Food for the Five Seasons: How Traditional Chinese Medicine Can Fuel Your Health

Christine Grisham, Dipl.OM, L.Ac., CMT, MA

Acknowledgements

I'd like to dedicate this book to anyone who struggles with health challenges. Keep pushing forward, and don't give up!

Thank you to my all of my beloved family and friends, who have listened to me talk these past few years about my own health struggles related to having a chronic autoimmune disease, and about the overwhelming details related to starting up a business.

I'm very grateful to my acupuncture patients for trusting me enough to be a part of such an intimate part of your lives. Thank you for working with me to improve your health and well-being.

Many thanks as well to all my professors at PCOM, especially Drs. Elizabeth Talcott, Gretchen Seitz da Silva and KC Conover. Special appreciation and thanks is reserved for Dr. Seitz da Silva for your generous advice and support throughout the years, and for helping to review the text of this book.

I owe appreciation and thanks to the people who helped edit and provide comments for this book, including my sister Colleen Grisham, and my compatriots April Joy Rodriguez, Jennifer McKeever, Lori Stephens, and Natalie Vail. I owe much of my recent successes to my business mastermind group members, Alice Olsher, Jeanne Burke, KishaLynn Elliott, and Shayla Logan. Special thanks is reserved for Anna Smith for your hard work, substantive input, and amazing editing skills.

Last, any factual errors are purely my own. Accurately representing a complex medical system that's thousands of years old is a heady task, and I hope that I have done it justice. A note to TCM practitioners and students: this book is meant as a primer for people who are largely unfamiliar with TCM and, out of necessity, some of the finer details of our medicine are not included. This is not intended to be a textbook!

Table of Contents

CHAPTER ONE: What This Book Can Do For You

This book will first introduce you to the idea that we need to connect nature's seasons, our bodies and our food in a meaningful way. Then, this book will guide you through the steps for how to create that connection in your life. In the process, the secrets behind an ancient, time-tested way of eating will be revealed (one that uses normal foods that are easy to get). Meals are simple and delicious, and will support your health based on your unique needs.

Have you ever asked yourself: "Why don't I feel good even though I'm doing everything "right"? Where can I find something that works for ME?" Perhaps you've stood in the grocery aisle, stared at shelves full of options, and felt totally lost about what to cook for dinner.

Maybe you're frustrated and confused by all the diet gimmicks out there. Diet trends try to seduce you. They make it sound like you can do just one thing for a short time and change your entire life. We've all probably fallen prey to one of these slick sales pitches:

- Want to have a flat tummy? Eat pounds of wheatgrass for the next seven days!
- Want to have bulging muscles? Drink this protein drink for the next month!

While these promises sound good, it's easy to see they are flawed. They aren't based on sound nutritional principles, and they won't provide the balance needed for overall good health. **Just as motors and engines must have the right kind of fuel to operate well, your body must also get the right amount and type of nutrients**. It needs the right mix of proteins, carbohydrates, fats, minerals, vitamins, and a host of other nutrients to function at its best.

But...you are busy! You have a LIFE to LIVE. You need simple, understandable food options. You need the options that work for YOU—because we're all unique. And there's not one single plan that works for every body—we all have different needs.

Maybe you're thinking: I've heard this all before. Here's another "expert" claiming that if I just eat this or that food, or do certain exercises, my health will magically improve. But what's missing from so many sales pitches is YOU. You are an INDIVIDUAL with specific needs, and you have an ability to help heal your own body. And it's easy to learn what YOUR UNIQUE needs are—by using the secrets of Traditional Chinese Medicine.

What is Traditional Chinese Medicine?
This book will introduce you to Traditional Chinese Medicine, the theory of the Five Phases and how you can use this ancient wisdom to eat great food and adopt healthier habits, *fueling your way to a better life. It's simple, straightforward information that you can easily adapt to your own style.*

For thousands of years, Traditional Chinese Medicine, or TCM for short, has had a balanced, holistic approach to health. It looks at each person's unique needs, honors nature and the seasons, and combines these things to balance the body.

The TCM way of looking at the world is very unlike the worldview of most of us raised in the West. Most likely, you grew up going to a Medical Doctor who treated you with drugs to relieve your symptoms when you were sick. The goal with TCM is to keep the body in balance with customized treatments in order to *prevent* illness. In ancient China, if you got sick, it meant your doctor had failed and he wouldn't get paid for treating you!

Almost all of TCM is foreign to us in the West. While we may have heard about "Yin and Yang", we may not know that those terms are all about health and balance in the body. Acupuncture is a big part of TCM, and many people have heard of it. But few have actually tried it or have any idea what it is like to get a treatment. **Most people are surprised to learn that TCM is a complete medical system, able to treat just about any modern health problem, and that it can often prevent illness.**

TCM gives power to each person by reminding us that we have an inborn ability to heal ourselves. In fact, acupuncture works by helping the body to heal itself by using its innate healing power. In other words, YOU are the most important part of the healing process: not drugs, and not your doctor.

TCM uses many ways to increase a person's health beyond acupuncture. Most acupuncturists also use herbal medicines, massage, diet and lifestyle to improve their patients' health. This works best when diet and lifestyle changes are made first, and acupuncture and herbs are used to reinforce these. **After all, acupuncture and herbal medicines won't keep us alive. But food is basic; it sustains us as living beings. If we eat well, good health will be a natural outcome. Eating well can also help prevent disease.**

Some of the terms and ideas in this book may be new to you. I ask that you just go with it—these theories and ways of living have been used for thousands of years, and by millions of people. (You can see the Resources chapter that list books describing the long history of TCM.) Anything that time-tested and proven obviously contains a lot of wisdom, and really works!

The wisdom of TCM is based on the knowledge of thousands of doctors. They watched and recorded what people ate, how they lived, and what happened to their health. One way they came to understand the human body was by comparing our health (and disease) to the changes in nature. This is known as the *Five Phase Theory*. In order to further explore TCM, it's important to first understand this theory.

What are the Five Phases?

The five phases represent the natural world. TCM practitioners often use the five phases (also called five elements or five stages) to help them diagnose and treat disease.

The five phases are:

Fire(火, *huŏ*)

Earth(土, *tŭ*)

Metal(金, *jīn*)

Water(水, *shuĭ*)

Wood(木, *mù*)

These five phases represent the circle of life, the movement between creation and destruction.

- *Fire* burns wood, and provides the heat and energy necessary for change and metabolism.
- *Earth* is created from the ash left after a fire and it provides the nourishment (enriched soil) for living things to flourish.
- *Metal* is formed from minerals within the earth.
- *Water* is needed for any life to begin, and when a seed is planted in earth and given water, it can grow into a tree (wood).
- *Wood* provides the fuel needed to create a fire.

Each of the five phases connects to its own:

- ***season of the calendar year***
- ***particular colors, especially of our fresh foods***
- ***internal organs in the human body***
- ***emotions that we feel (in healthy ways and unbalanced ways).***

Throughout the book, I'll discuss each of these and how you can use this information to fuel your health and diet by making easy and positive changes in your life.

CHAPTER TWO: Identifying Your Unique Seasonal Style

How do the Five Phases relate to my health?

Each phase corresponds to two major organs that share similar functions and actions:

Fire relates to the Heart and its paired organ the Small Intestine. The Heart is in charge of blood circulation as well as thinking and brain power. The Small Intestine helps drain excess fire (heat) from the body, and rid the body of waste.

Earth relates to the Spleen and its paired organ the Stomach. The Stomach starts to break down and move food through the body. The Spleen changes food into usable nutrients for the body, helping to produce blood and control the muscles.

Metal relates to the Lungs and their paired organ the Large Intestine. The Lungs control the movement of air, energy, and water through the body (mainly the upper body), even out to our skin. The Large Intestine helps take excess waste and fluids out of the body.

Water relates to the Kidneys and their paired organ the Urinary Bladder. Both relate to moving fluids out of the body, but the Kidneys are also important in growth, development and reproduction.

Wood relates to the Liver and its paired organ the Gallbladder. The Liver controls the tendons and ligaments, stores blood and keeps the energy of the body flowing properly. The Gallbladder stores and excretes bile. Both organs help people maintain their emotions.

You'll notice that the functions of the organs are often quite similar to the actions of the five phases in nature (described in Chapter One). You may also see that many of the organs' functions differ from what you may have learned in anatomy classes in school. This is a good example of how the story of the human body can be interpreted (and correctly) in more than one way. TCM theories about anatomy and the human body are highly developed and have been tested on real people for thousands of years. In fact, many texts still being used today, including those related to diagnosis of disease, herbal medicines, and acupuncture treatments, were actually written over 2,000 years ago!

Why is it important to connect these theories to my life and diet?

My purpose for writing this book is that you will learn a new way of thinking about your health, your body, how to be more connected to nature and the seasons and what foods will fuel your body's health.

All too often, we are either sitting inside, closed up inside our home, workplace, or car. It's easy to be totally disconnected from nature, barely feeling the sun on our skin or breathing fresh air. Instead, our air temperature and lights are carefully controlled and, for all we know, it could be any time of year. *We need to get back to a more natural existence* and one way to do this is to know more about our own individual needs and characteristics, by using the cycle of nature's seasons to better-understand ourselves. To do this, I've taken ancient TCM theories and developed what I call Seasonal Styles.

What is a "Seasonal Style"? How do I identify mine?

A Seasonal Style combines the wisdom of TCM theory with modern living. There are five Seasonal Styles, which correspond to each of the five phases recognized by TCM.

You're probably wondering—aren't there *four* seasons every year? In *five phase* theory, the "fifth" season is known as early fall or harvest time, basically the transition from summer into fall. It relates to the Spleen and Stomach, which are both digestive organs in TCM. Connecting harvest time with the Spleen/Stomach makes sense, as the body's digestive system nourishes the body and early fall is when we harvest our food from the fields.

Each season has a unique impact on our lives. *Summer* is hot and muggy and can be a time of great fun and joyful outdoor activities. During the *early fall*, plants are returning to the ground, helping to nourish the soil for next year and we are often reminded of the bounty of harvest and enjoy many yummy, healthy foods that are hard to find at other times. In the *autumn*, things are further dying off and transitioning into the cold of winter, which can make us long for (grieve) the nice summer weather. During *winter*, most of us retreat to the protection of the indoors and, like the proverbial hibernating bear, we spend more time resting and engaging in quieter activities. Last, we move to *spring*, with much new growth and a return to full activity, which can feel quite chaotic. And then the cycle begins again.

Five phase theory suggests that most people are born with a body type that mirrors one the five phases (seasons). As a result, each person tends to have nutritional needs, health problems, and even a personality type that correspond to "their season". What I hope becomes clear to you is that these theories are so powerful because you can use them to improve your health in a natural way.

To help you understand which of the five Seasonal Styles represents you best, I have developed a **Seasonal Style Symptom Indicator**, a quick and easy worksheet that can be completed in about 20 minutes. (See the attached Appendix for the *Indicator*.) Please give this worksheet careful consideration, as it can be a helpful guide in improving your overall well-being.

Note: *it is common to fall into more than one Seasonal Style*. There are many possible reasons for this: you may lead a very busy, stressful life. You may suffer from chronic health issues. Perhaps your diet isn't ideal, you don't get enough sleep, or exercise very regularly. Life stages like puberty, menopause, pregnancy, or childbirth can affect your Seasonal Style. In addition, significant life changes like the beginning of a relationship, moving to a different climate, changing jobs, or the death of a loved one can also affect your health and lead you to have health symptoms relating to more than one Seasonal Style.

If you do find that you're checking symptoms in multiple Seasonal Style categories on the Symptom Indicator, don't be alarmed. This is likely just a reflection of the many stresses and demands of modern life. You may ultimately need to identify with more than one Seasonal Style. And if you fall into more than one Seasonal Style, even if one is dominant, I recommend buying any and all chapters that correspond to your symptoms so you'll learn about any Seasonal Styles that apply directly to you, and so that you get a more holistic picture of the theories presented here.

And guess what? *If it's the time of year on the calendar that corresponds to your particular Seasonal Style, the health issues that you commonly experience are likely to be worse.* This is one very important reason for you to know what Seasonal Style fits you best: so that you can be prepared for your upcoming season. I'm a Winter/ Water phase, so I know to begin taking particular herbs and eating a lot of warming, dark foods (like red beans, soups and meat) a month or two before we move into wintertime. Otherwise, my body temperature feels freezing and I have a sore back and knees.

It's also important to know that even if you don't match up with a particular Seasonal Style, you may have health symptoms and needs matching that Style during its particular season. Maybe you're not a water person like me. Yet you may actually have water-related symptoms during the winter. For example, it's helpful for *everyone* to rest more during winter, and especially so if you feel more run-down than usual.

I completed the checklist and now I know my Seasonal Style. Now what?

Once you've completed the Seasonal Style Symptom Checklist and identified your unique Style (or Styles), you'll most likely wonder: "So what? Now what do I do with this information?" Knowing which Seasonal Style fits you best can help you address current health concerns and stay balanced and healthy in the long run. ***The food you take in, the way you live and how you balance the inevitable stresses and emotions of life can all relate to your dominant Seasonal Style. Remember these three words and you're halfway home:***

- ***FOOD***
- ***LIFESTYLE***
- ***EMOTIONS***

Food

So you're standing in the grocery store and thinking "What am I going to buy today? I'm so tired of planning meals!" It can feel draining and time consuming to plan meals all the time. Or even worse, you just give up, leave the store and instead buy whatever takeout happens to suit your fancy that day.

An easy and quick shortcut for your grocery list is to **focus on the *colors* of the fresh foods you're buying**. You may be aware that when a food is a particular color, this indicates it has certain vitamins and minerals. But specific colors also support the Seasonal Styles:

Fire is red
Earth is yellow and orange
Metal is white
Water is blue and black
Wood is green

Say for example that you have completed the Seasonal Style Symptom Checklist. It's clear you identify most with the phase Wood, because you have symptoms such as difficult menstrual cycles, often feel irritable and short-tempered, and have very tight muscles. By eating more green foods like kale and spinach, you can fuel the energy of your Liver and, over time, help improve your symptoms. This same principle applies to all five Seasonal Styles—once you identify which one you are, you can choose more foods with the season's matching color to help improve your health. It's that simple!

In addition to the color of foods, **it's also helpful to pay attention to the action fresh foods have on your body once you eat them**. This may be a totally new idea to you, but it can affect your health in important ways. In particular, the *temperature* of a food is very important.

Temperature boils down to (no pun intended) whether the food has a warming or cooling effect on the body; some foods have a neutral effect on body temperature. Warming foods tend to provide more calories, revving up the body and they are often animal products. Cooling foods usually have a slowing-down effect on the body, with high concentrations of water, less calories and tend to be

fruits or vegetables. (Note that the temperature of a food is about how it affects your body, not necessarily if you have actually cooked or chilled it.)

Common symptoms of too much heat in the body include: a feeling of warm body temperature, a desire for cold drinks and foods, agitation/ irritation, excessive sweating, high blood pressure, and constipation. Common symptoms of too much cold in the body include: chilly sensations, a desire for warm foods and drinks, cold hands and feet, wanting to wear many layers of clothes and pains that are cramping and fixed.

If you have symptoms that show you have too much heat in your body, it can help if you eat more cooling foods. Likewise, if you have too much cold, you should eat more warming foods. Depending on your Seasonal Style and current health challenges, you likely will need a bit more of foods with either hot or cold temperatures. This concept of food and temperature will be explained further in the five Seasonal Style chapters.

Lifestyle

The dreaded word "lifestyle". Often it sounds so vague and even accusatory. What does this really mean? It really comes down to how we spend our day: how much do we move? how much do we express our true selves? do we have a career that uplifts our spirit? do we engage in risky behaviors that hurt us in the long run, although they're fun today? do we have a sense of balance between having fun and our responsibilities?

A huge factor among all of the questions listed above is how we deal with stress and emotions. Each of the five Seasonal Styles has unique lifestyle components that are explored in the following chapters.

Emotions

If you have mental health struggles such as anxiety, depression, fear, or anger, I doubt you've ever heard that your symptoms will likely be worse during a specific season. In Traditional Chinese Medicine, each season is associated with a particular emotion, influencing a specific part of the body's energetic system and organs and thus aggravating particular physical health issues, too.

We all know that there are normal, healthy levels of emotions, as well as emotions that are unbalanced and uncontrolled. The five phases are paired with emotions in this way:
   Fire relates to joy.
   Earth relates to worry or excessive thinking.

Metal relates to sadness and grief.
Water relates to fear.
Wood relates to anger.

Feelings are a part of life. But sometimes we can lose our balance and begin to feel a certain emotion too deeply, too strongly. Over time, this affects our physical health because the matching organ system also becomes unbalanced. (For instance, let's say you worry a lot about your family and work so much that you really overexert your brain. Over time, this affects your Earth phase, and you will likely develop digestive problems.)

Having unbalanced emotions can be a vicious cycle: you feel too much, so your body works less efficiently and vice versa. But, we can stop this process by being aware of what's going on, and correct our diet and lifestyle choices so that we support whatever organ system has become out of whack.

My Unique Seasonal Style + Food + Lifestyle + Emotions = ?

Taken all together, once you have identified your Seasonal Style and read the appropriate chapters in this book, you will know more about how to:

- Identify the signs and symptoms that show you're out of balance
- Gauge your health by the five phases
- Empower yourself to take charge of your own health
- Reduce your chronic health struggles (pain, sleeping problems, poor digestion and more!)
- Know what types of foods to eat and what lifestyle habits to adopt
- Reinvent your grocery list

Tips for reading *Food for the Five Seasons*
First, read the first two chapters in order to understand the basics. Second, complete the *Seasonal Style Symptom Indicator* and identify which of the five Seasonal Styles matches you best. Then, either purchase the chapter that matches your Seasonal Style, or purchase the entire book to get the additional bonus chapters.

Having the entire book will give you a great reference for your entire family, as you may fit into differing Seasonal Styles. In addition, even if you don't fit into a particular Seasonal Style, adapting some of the foods and lifestyle habits that go with a season during that particular season will help keep you balanced and healthy in general.

Chapters Three through Seven describe each of the five Seasonal Styles in more detail. In each chapter, you'll learn more about its Seasonal Style and be provided ***examples of what foods to eat, exercise and lifestyle recommendations, how to increase your emotional health, as well as a sample grocery checklist.***

Chapter Eight is a bonus chapter on dealing with excess body weight from the TCM perspective. *Chapter Nine* summarizes the book and *Chapter 10* provides a few resources for more reading.

Again, my hope and goal for writing this book is for you as a reader to adopt the knowledge provided by these ancient theories, so that you can truly improve your health while also living more in harmony with nature and the passing seasons.

What if I want to learn more about TCM and the Five Phases?
If you would like more guidance and advice that what I've given here, I've listed several resources by other authors in

Chapter 10. In addition, I also strongly recommend that you seek the care of a licensed acupuncturist. Licensed acupuncturists have Master of Science degrees, typically with over 3,000 hours of training in subjects like Chinese medical theory, clinical counseling and Western anatomy and physiology. Many are also trained in prescribing herbal medicine. Licensed acupuncturists are also trained as general practitioners and can thus improve many health problems, help you maintain your health and assist you in making diet and lifestyle changes—and in a *much* more in-depth manner than this book could ever possibly cover.

Remember, TCM is thousands of years old, with knowledge based on extensive clinical evidence. A capable practitioner is able to improve almost any health issue you can imagine, be it physical, emotional, or even spiritual. The beauty and strength of TCM is that its vast knowledge base is used to treat your specific condition for that specific day. So go find a licensed acupuncturist! A good start is searching the websites Acufinder.com or TCMDirectory.com.

Last, the information here is _not_ intended to be a substitute for medical advice, diagnosis or treatment from a trained and licensed health care provider. Please consult a licensed health care professional before embarking on any major diet or lifestyle change.

CHAPTER THREE: THE FIRE PHASE

Imagine a hot summer night. You're on vacation for two weeks and you've taken a trip to a beautiful cabin. You're feeling an amorous passion for your sweetie. It's almost like a cartoon, where your big, red heart leaps outside of your chest with joy when you see her/him walk into the room. Quite an image, yes? This scene contains the general qualities of the fire phase: *our Heart, joyful emotions, summertime, hot weather and the color red.*

The important role of the Heart in the body: Not just blood circulation!
Fire relates to the *Heart* and its paired organ the Small Intestine. The Heart is in charge of making the blood, conscious thinking and brain power. It is also said to "house" the spirit-mind, or *Shen*. The *Shen* is both the soul and mental consciousness. In other words, having a healthy Heart is more than just a physical thing related to the blood vessels.

In TCM, the Heart is also thought to drain excess heat from the body via its relationship with the Small Intestine, which excretes waste from the body. Draining out that extra heat is a good thing, because if you have excess heat in the Heart, you become unbalanced and the normal feeling of joy morphs into manic behavior. You can have signs such as very frequent, loud and even inappropriate laughter, anxiety and insomnia (mainly difficulty falling asleep). Some people have so much heat in their Heart that it rises to their head and they get canker sores in their mouths!

Here are other common heat symptoms for people with the Fire/Heart Seasonal Style: racing heart or palpitations, chest pains and other mental/emotional problems like confused thinking, feeling scared easily, or even serious mental illness. These symptoms can be more pronounced than usual during the summer months.

On the completely opposite end of the spectrum, sometimes a person has *too little Fire*, or basically what's called Heart *Qi* and *Yang* deficiency, which is a lack of Heart energy with too much cold. Symptoms here can include: hardened arteries, angina (severe chest pain), nervousness, depression, and lethargy.

The fun of it: maintain that joyful balance
You may be thinking: "These symptoms don't sound too fun… what happened to all the joy"? Joy is the normal, harmonious emotion connected with the Heart. But when the Heart gets out of balance, people lose their joy and tend to go to an

extreme. As I mentioned above, they may have manic behaviors, or go the opposite way and feel depressed.
TCM texts talk about several ways to help maintain a healthy Heart balance and these tips aren't common knowledge. For starters, remember the Shen, or spirit-mind? Yes, keeping our veins and arteries clear of junk is very important, but how about keeping one's SPIRITS squeaky clean? You can aid Heart health by calming your mind. One way to do this is by using your voice, such as by talking about a stressful day with a friend or family member. You can also help the spirit relax and feel more harmonious by doing activities that calm and center you. Meditation, prayer, chanting and affirmations are just a few examples. These help heal our Heart by more fully integrating our spirit and thoughts.

But what if you have *too little* passion and feel depressed? What does it look like? If you have what TCM calls heart "deficiency", it looks somewhat like it sounds. You may have a weak pulse, body weakness and a cold feeling in your body; you may be depressed or feel lethargic or tired. If you have

25

this type of deficiency, eating red foods to build up your heart energy and the amount of blood in your body can really help (see more below on food recommendations).

Sweltering summer: sweat a little!
Since **Summer** is the time for hot weather, we need to be sure to keep our Heart balanced by having enough fluids in the body so that we don't overheat. This is important because, as mentioned above, the Heart houses the *Shen* (mental cognition and spirit) and also is in charge of circulating the blood. If the body overheats, this agitates the mind and one can feel that the "blood is boiling"!

But before you eat that big bowl of ice cream, be careful! It's much more beneficial to your body to sweat a little instead and cool off naturally. It may sound counterintuitive, but drinking warm liquids, eating a bit of spicy food and taking hot showers will help you to cool down. So be careful with those big glasses of iced drinks and huge, raw salads! They make your system too cold and your digestive organs will work less effectively. Hot chrysanthemum or mint teas are great options. But balance is the key—avoid taking in large amounts of anything that's too hot OR too cold.

Fueling foods for the Heart: cooling the fire
When eating foods to help balance the fire phase, think **RED, COOLING and FLUIDS.** Red foods are great to eat because they nourish the Heart and build up the blood supply in the body. Experiment and have fun—include the lesser-known types of fruits and berries like hawthorn berry, or Schisandrae fruit, which you'll find at Asian food stores. (More on these Chinese herbs in the Grocery list at the end of the chapter).

Other great foods to eat during summer include: celery, cucumber and lettuce are cooling and support the healthy functioning of the Heart. Fruits like apples, lemon, lime and watermelon also help beat the heat. Mushrooms and high quality whole grains like brown rice and oats are very calming for the *Shen*.

Get creative with cooking. The great part about summer is that it's the best time of year to get fresh produce in an array of dazzling colors. Add some spice to that beautiful produce and cook your food quickly. Stir fries are great this time of year.

Foods that drain the Heart energy
Avoid heavy, greasy, oily and fatty foods and overeating in general. Limit your intake of meat and eggs, especially any-thing processed. It can be easy to forget, but eating light in summer is natural and helps the system to reboot.

Lifestyle ideas: *get busy living*
In general, summer is a time of abundance everywhere you look. It's a great time of year to be fully engaged in life. Work hard, vacation hard, serve your community, visit with friends and family: go full force! Get up early and use your creativity to its fullest. *Enjoy* the abundant nature of summertime: have fun with the extra sunlight hours and energy provided by this time of year!

However, check in with yourself often and be REALLY honest: are you feeling depressed and withdrawing from life? Are you manic and is your mind all over the place? If either situation is happening for you, you may need help from a professional. I also recommend that you take time to practice calming activi-ties that soothe your spirit. (See the comments on *Shen* above.)

The Western biomedical perspective
Red foods have been shown to support Heart health. Many red foods contain antioxidants, which reduce free radicals in

the body. Free radicals have been shown to increase the damage or even cause death to healthy cells in the body, which is an important issue for blood vessels and Heart health. Tomatoes have lycopene, a powerful antioxidant that helps prevent Heart disease. Red bell peppers also contain lycopene, as well as potassium, which can help lower elevated blood pressure. Red grapes have been shown to lower blood pressure, reduce inflammation and reduce Heart muscle damage related to a high-salt diet. Tart red cherries contain anthocyanins, powerful antioxidants that help reduce inflammation (good for problems such as arthritis and gout) and they have Heart-health benefits.

Take Away Message
  Food- Red colors, full of fluid, with cooling properties
 Lifestyle- Be active and engaged but take time to quiet your mind
 Emotion- Do what makes you feel joyful and spend time with happy people

Fire/ Heart Seasonal Style Grocery List
Red foods:
Red peppers
Tomatoes
Raspberries, strawberries
Red grapes
Tart cherries

Cooling foods with high fluid content:
Celery
Cucumber
Lettuce
Apples
Lemon and lime
Watermelon

To relax the mind:
Mushrooms
High quality whole grains like brown rice, oat and wheat

Cooling drinks (use in moderation):
Mint, chrysanthemum, and chamomile teas

To clear heat from the body (also use in moderation):
Black Pepper
Cayenne pepper
Fresh Ginger
Hot peppers

Chinese herbs:
NOTE: While many Chinese herbs are also foods, it's important to consult with a TCM practitioner before consuming more than a minimal amount of these products, as a professional will provide you with the proper dosages as well as how to prepare them. (The English, Latin and Chinese names are provided to help you shop more easily for them.)

- Hawthorn berries (Latin Crataegi Fructus, Chinese Shan Zha)—moves the blood and helps improve hypertension and elevated cholesterol.
- Dragon Eye or Longan fruit (Latin Longan Arillus, Chinese Long Yan Rou)—builds the Heart blood and relaxes the mind.
- Jujube seeds (Latin Ziziphus spinosa, Chinese Da Zao)—helps relax the mind.
- Schisandrae fruit (Latin name Schisandrae Fructus, Chinese Wu Wei Zi)—helps relax the mind.

CHAPTER FOUR: THE EARTH PHASE

It's an early morning near the end of summer as a farmer harvests his mature, yellow corn crop. It's hot and humid for this time of year, but he's pleased anyway because it's been a bountiful season. This year, unlike in some past years, the farmer doesn't have to worry too much that his hard efforts working to feed other people will also in return help him feed his own family. Inside his family's home, his wife is cooking a special meal. Unlike her husband, she's been worrying constantly for weeks: their only child is about to leave for college. She's hoping that serving their child's favorite meal of chicken and fresh butternut squash will help their daughter remember how much they love her. This scene describes our focus of this chapter: *the Spleen and digestion, late summer and harvest time, worry (or pensiveness) and foods that are yellow or orange in color.*

The Spleen's important role in our bodies: Digest food, absorb nutrients!

Earth relates to the *Spleen* and its paired organ the Stomach. These organs change our food into usable nutrients for the body, helping to make blood and control the muscles. In TCM, the Stomach is responsible for the initial breaking down of "grain and water" (i.e., food). The Spleen then extracts the essence of grain and water (the nutrients contained in the food) and sends it to the other organs in the body. Last, note that what TCM views as the Spleen includes the functions of the pancreas. The pancreas aids in digestion through the actions of enzymes, and it plays a vital role in helping the body utilize glucose (sugar).

The Earth phase is so foundational to your body that you should think of it as your *center.* (Well, it is actually located in the middle of your body, but you know what I mean!) The Spleen and the digestive system is truly the hub of life, the beginning step for all of your body's activity, as it provides the basic materials used by all the other organs.

When our Earth phase is not working at its best, the basic nutrients we need to have energy and be active in our lives are missing. Signs of this are: fatigue, lack of physical strength and lack of mental awareness. Digestive problems are common and include gas, bloating, nausea, poor appetite or getting hungry soon after eating, acid reflux and loose stools. You may have blood sugar issues and struggle with being overweight, yet do not eat much. Or you may be very thin and cannot gain weight. A lack of Earth phase balance can also show up as being prone to worry a lot, and perhaps not being able to maintain a tidy home or appearance because you may lack the energy to maintain order in general.

A word about mucus...
Oh, Spleen. You're so hard-working but terribly under-appreciated! Much like Mother Earth is the foundation of our natural world, providing us sustenance and giving life, we wouldn't be alive without our own internal Earth organs. The workings of the entire digestive system (Spleen/ Stomach/ Pancreas/ Intestines) must be healthy in order for us to function well. However... **the modern American diet causes our bodies to create a lot of mucus, or "damp"**. We eat refined, processed, boxed, bagged, bleached "food" that often has little or no nutritional value. (More on this in Chapter Eight regarding excess weight.)

Picture a runny nose, but all over the inside of your body! This damp/ mucus can lead to severe problems in our bodies. In order to stop the damp, we must first and foremost address the digestive system. People with too much mucus tend to be overweight, but don't eat much. They often have swelling (edema) in their joints or abdomen, and digestive problems such as poor appetite, loose bowel movements and nausea. And they may also have a feeling of a heavy body, especially their head and limbs, and can feel "stuck" in their lives. People with too much mucus also commonly have a "fuzzy feeling" mentally.

Some of the best foods for those with Earth Seasonal Style help nourish the digestive system and/or help reduce the amount of mucus in the body. (Foods to dry dampness in the body are listed in the Grocery List at the end of the chapter.) These foods to reduce dampness are important because keeping mucus at a balanced level is vital. Mucus not only affects our digestion, it can also lead to problems in other organs. Mucus can affect the Heart and Lungs, and plays a role in such problems as allergies, stuffy noses, and even mental health problems. Our digestive organs are our "center" and we have to work to keep them running at full capacity!

The Earth is your center: the source of your body's stability

People often strive to be "grounded." They say you should "trust your gut." The earth under our feet is our literal "foundation." Although it may sound a little far-fetched to think that all of these common sayings are closely tied to the health of our digestive organs, it is true. When the body isn't fed correctly, the spirit can't flourish. When your Spleen is unbalanced, you may worry too much over things you can't control, or about things that may not be that important in the big scheme of life. Hopefully by now, you can see how feeding your "center" properly keeps you stable and from becoming "off center" and thus unhealthy!

Worry, also known as pensiveness, is the hallmark of the person with a deficient Spleen. Think of the people you know who eat when they feel stressed—perhaps it's you. They have repetitive, intrusive and unhelpful thoughts about work, family, whatever—and they comfort themselves by running to the fridge for a sweet snack. They often also have trouble falling asleep because their worries repeatedly run through their minds as they lie in bed.

Finding better ways to feed your body (therefore your soul) is without question vital to breaking the cycle of constant worry. It starts with diet, but it's really about how you choose to create balance *everywhere* in your life, especially by creating a regular schedule and habits. (More on schedules when we get to the section on Lifestyle Ideas!)

Nourishing harmony and balance during change and transition

The **Earth** phase is about **early fall**, around the last month of summer when the farmer harvests and prepares his fields for winter. It's the time when the abundance of spring and summer moves towards the time of more quiet, inward activities. Here the focus should be on balance and peacefulness in the face of change—even more than at other times of the year.

But the Earth phase is also about transition in general, not just at one time of year. **The Earth is special because it can be associated with the transitions between *ALL of the seasons* of the year**—both the week before and the week following each new season. Eating foods supporting the Spleen throughout the year, especially as we transition between seasons, can help you effectively deal with changes in your life and keep you feeling healthier.

Change is hard for just about all of us, in part because we like what's known; it's a lot easier to understand what's already in front of us. A concept from Taoism and the more modern Aesop's fables comes to mind: an oak bracing itself against the wind will blow over, but the reed that bends, adapts and adjusts will survive the storm. Life is not static—nothing remains the same. This is a given. In order to be healthy, we must learn ways to adapt. Being unyielding, unbending, rigid and stiff is akin to an early death!

Fueling foods for the Spleen: *cultivate your belly health, dry the mucus*

Improving any symptoms that relate to the Earth phase are absolutely tied to your diet: making better food choices is *the most important change* you can make to improve your health. So how do you "cultivate" your belly health? The wording here is intentional. When you shop for fresh foods that nourish your Earth phase, think of a garden in autumn, which needs a bit of cultivation and care to flourish. In the garden, you'll find lots of hearty yellow and orange foods like squash, carrots and pumpkin. Foods that harmonize and support the digestive organs and those that help drain any excess damp/mucus are best; see the grocery list at the end of the chapter for more ideas.

When you eat your meals, focus on the deliciousness of the food itself, so add few spices or oil to your food, especially during the autumn. Let the natural flavors of these hearty foods shine through. You can cook what's known as a *congee* soup, a creamy and slow-cooked rice porridge. (See the end of this chapter for a recipe.) Congee, the ultimate comfort food, is very effective after an illness, especially stomach flu, and is a great option for infants because their digestive systems aren't fully mature.

Foods that drain the Spleen energy

Some foods tend to tax our digestive organs, often leading to excess damp in our bodies. If you are an Earth Seasonal Style, you are particularly prone to damp and need to pay attention. And for everyone, eating too much of damp-causing foods will eventually damage the digestive organs. But... it's important to eat *some* of these foods in moderation because they do contain nutrients that your body needs. (This is an area in which an acupuncturist or similar practitioner can help you tailor your food choices as you seek to maximize your health.)

Some examples of foods that tend to put stress on the digestive organs and thus should be eaten in moderation include: citrus fruits and juices, tomatoes, sugars (honey, corn syrup, molasses), dairy products like milk and butter, wheat, alcohol, cooking oils, nuts and seeds, and animal proteins like meat and eggs. Dairy and sugar in particular are huge culprits in the creation of too much mucus in the body. (Think cookies, breads and pasta.)

In addition, eating too many greasy, fried foods and alcohol can cause a buildup of **too much heat** in the digestive organs, particularly the Stomach, leading to symptoms like headaches on the forehead, burping and heartburn.

On the other hand, one major way to *improve* your belly's health is to keep it from getting **too cold**. Cold drinks and foods, like raw green salads or iced drinks are hard for your Spleen and Stomach to digest and over time make those organs weak. Too many cold foods can create cramping in the abdomen, as well as also lead to menstrual problems in women because the Liver is affected over the long-term (it's in charge of the movement of blood). Foods that cool the body and are especially tough on the digestive organs include seaweed, spinach, tofu and tomato.

Ice cream is ultimate example of a food that taxes the Spleen and Stomach! It's cold, made of animal protein, very sweet and is often full of unnatural preservatives. Pizza is another great example: acidic tomato sauce, cheese, greasy meat and wheat are all known to increase the damp in your body. Watch out for those disaster foods!

Lifestyle Ideas: *trust and respect your gut's "time clock"*
Here is a list of habits of suggestions to adopt if you wish to improve your Earth/ Spleen health. Compared to other Seasonal Styles, the list a bit longer and I would argue more important. Why is this? Remember, having a healthy digestive system is the basis of our health, it is our center.

Many of these habits relate to **having a regular schedule**. Many of us want to do this. However, it can be very difficult to maintain healthy habits. I assure you, it is vital to make a regular schedule a part of your life. In fact, this is one of the single most important things you can do to improve your health. (If you'd like even more tips on how to do this, see Chapter 8 on excess weight.)

- Focus on peaceful, thoughtful mealtimes. Make it a joyful event with your loved ones. It's not a time to continue the fight you're currently having with your partner, or for doing other activities such as watching the newest (and violent!) cop show on TV.
- Eat at the same times every day. Your digestive system needs and thrives on regularity. (They don't refer to bowel movement "regularity" by accident!) This also helps you maintain a relatively level amount of sugar, or glucose, in your blood.
- Chew each bite thoroughly. Digestion begins in the mouth with the amylase enzyme in your saliva. Thorough chewing also helps you focus on the beauty and gift of the meal.
- Don't eat large meals close to bedtime. This diverts the energy (*qi*) needed for repairing the body back into the digestive system. As a result, you aren't able to properly heal and rest and you can also suffer from insomnia.
- Avoid eating too much food at one time because large meals burden the digestion. (think how you feel after Thanksgiving dinner!)
- Prepare for sleep. During the last hour of the day, engage in quiet, relaxing activities and turn of all lighted

screens (TV, phone, tablet, laptop, Kindle, etc.) Keep the same bedtime and rise at the same time every day. This will help create a peaceful atmosphere, quieting your mind and helping prevent sleepless nights where you lie awake with repetitive thoughts running through your mind like an endless loop.

- Exercise! We all know this, but one motivation that may be new to you is that exercise is needed to keep damp mucus from building up in your body. Walking is an excellent way to begin. You **do not** need to burn thousands of calories or work out for hours at a time at the gym in order to benefit from exercise.
- Practice abdominal self-massage. If you have constipation or diarrhea, self-massage is a subtle message to send your body. It helps balance your digestion and elimination. (You can easily find information about how to do this online.)
- Create a general routine in your life so that your body knows what to expect, but don't be so rigid that you can't respond to the larger, more important changes that are bound to happen (see the oak and the reed story described above).

Western biomedical perspective

Yellow fruits and vegetables contain carotenoids and bioflavonoids, which are a class of water soluble plant pigments that function as antioxidants. Along with antioxidants, yellow foods also have a lot of vitamin C. These nutrients help your Heart, vision, digestion and immune system.

Orange foods often contain Vitamin A and beta carotene. Beta carotene is a powerful antioxidant. It is good for eye health, can delay cognitive aging and protect the skin from sun damage. Beta carotene is a precursor for vitamin A, which is important for night vision. It also can neutralize free radicals in the body, which is crucial to the health of your immune system, and a majority of your immune cells are located in your digestive system.

Eating oranges or orange juice is not advised for people who have excess damp, but other people can eat them in moderation without problems. Eat citrus foods whole when possible (not juiced, unless it's a small amount of fresh-squeezed). Oranges are among the few foods that contain a large amount of soluble fiber, which moderates increases in blood glucose levels and reduces buildup of cholesterol. Other benefits of fiber include increasing feelings of fullness after eating, and aiding the intestinal immune system. Oranges may help to prevent certain cancers, particularly of the stomach. Oranges also contain thiamine. (A word of caution: go easy on the amount of acidic foods you ingest including foods like oranges and tomatoes, because they can aggravate your Stomach and cause heartburn.)

Take Away Message

Food- Yellow and orange colored, hearty rice porridges, but limit the damp foods
Lifestyle- Create a regular schedule but stay flexible and adjust to change
Emotion- Don't let yourself fall into pensive, worrisome thoughts—take action

Earth/ Spleen Seasonal Style Grocery List

Yellow and orange foods to harmonize the center:
Carrots
Pumpkin
Squash (summer, yellow, winter)
Sweet potato
Tofu
Yellow pepper
Apricots
Bananas
Cantaloupe
Kumquat
Lemons
Mango
Oranges
Papaya
Peaches
Plantain
Pineapple
Star Fruit

Some foods to harmonize the digestive system:
Beans (garbanzo, soy, string)
Cabbage
Corn
Grains (amaranth, rice)
Chestnuts

Some foods to help reduce damp mucus:
Celery
Corn
Lettuce
Pumpkin
Scallion
Grains like amaranth, rice and rye
Azuki beans (also known as aduki)
Raw honey
Goat's milk products (as a substitute for the usual cow's milk)

Chinese herbs:
NOTE: While many Chinese herbs are also foods, it's important to consult with a TCM practitioner before consuming more
than a minimal amount of these products, as a professional
will provide you with the proper dosages as well as how to
prepare them. (The English, Latin and Chinese names are
provided to help you shop more easily for them.)

- Cardamon fruit (Latin Amomi Fructus, Chinese Sha
  Ren and Bai Dou Kou)—slightly warms the digestive
  organs and helps stop diarrhea due to cold.
- Hyacinth bean (Latin Lablab semen, Chinese Bai Bian
  Dou)—strengthens Spleen, reduces damp, warms the
  digestive organs.

Congee Recipe (very simple!)

Rice (Latin Oryzae Semen, Chinese Geng Mi) is used as a
medicinal herb in TCM, helping to nourish the digestive organs, stop diarrhea and reduce excess damp/ mucus in the
body. It's especially helpful for young children and people recovering from a long-term or serious illness.

Ingredients (Serves 6 to 8):
3/4 cup long grain or brown rice
9 cups water
1 teaspoon salt

Preparation: In a large pot, bring the water and rice to a boil.
When the rice is boiling, turn the heat down to medium low.
Place the lid on the pot and tilt it open slightly to allow steam
to escape. Continue cooking on medium low or low heat, stir-
ring occasionally, until the rice has the thick, creamy texture of
porridge (cook time is usually about 1 hour). Once done, add
the salt to taste, and any other seasonings if desired.

Feel free to add other ingredients to this recipe such as meat,
fish, and vegetables. Add these secondary ingredients after
bringing the rice to a boil, when you turn down the heat. The

key is to cook the rice so that it's a creamy texture, because your goal is a dish that's easy to digest and absorb.

CHAPTER FIVE: THE METAL PHASE

It's a chilly fall day and as you walk along the sidewalk, you hear the crunch of dead leaves under your feet. You take a deep breath and feel the crisp, cold air pass through your nostrils, down to your Lungs. You gaze up to the tree line and see that the leaves are quickly losing their color, drying up, and falling through the air to the ground below. Everything is starting to look almost white as winter approaches. Nature is contracting, turning inward and downward. As you walk, you think about the nature of autumn, and feel a bit sad that another year is complete and that the beauty and abundance of summer is ending. But you also know that this transition is necessary. Soon it will be winter, white snow will cover the ground, life will slow down, and the plants that are now dying and returning to the group will provide the nourishment for new ones to bloom and flourish in the spring. This scene helps describe our focus of this chapter: ***the Lungs and breath, autumn, the emotion grief and foods that are white or light-colored.***

The Lungs' important role in our bodies: Gate to our world!

Metal relates to the Lungs and their paired organ the Large Intestine. The Lungs regulate the movement of air, energy, and fluids through the body (mainly the upper body), even out to the skin where the pores open and close. The Large Intestine helps take excess waste and fluids out of the body, cleansing the body of unhealthy toxins.

Together, the Lungs, Large Intestine, and skin provide our immune barrier against the outside world. If you think about it, the Lungs are the only internal organs that are exposed to the outside world! Each time you breathe, you take in a bit of the world around you. So, it's important to keep your Lungs strong in order to have the best health possible because they play such a big part in disease resistance. In TCM, the Lungs relate directly to the skin and control the pores, and this is part of how they help keep our immunity strong. The skin's pores act like tiny Lungs: they open to help us sweat and cleanse the body, and close to keep out harmful germs. If you have robust Lungs, you recover quickly from illnesses, your skin and complexion are bright, and your voice is clear and strong.

People with weak Lungs are often physically weak with poor vitality and immunity. Their breathing may be shallow; perhaps they suffer from problems such as allergies, asthma, bronchitis and frequent colds. Their skin may look unhealthy, dry and splotchy, because the flow of *Qi* (or energy) and fluids in their body is poor. They may also have problems with their Intestines and have abnormal bowel movements. People with weak Lungs tend to suffer from lingering sadness and low self-esteem. They also may struggle with proper boundaries, and tend to harshly judge both themselves and others.

Other health symptoms related to weak Lungs can be divided into three groups: Lung dryness, Lung phlegm, and deficient Lung Qi.

- *Lung dryness* leads to dryness of the skin, face, and throat, as well as itching. Dryness is often a result of weather and is made worse by indoor heaters during the colder months. Dryness can lead to too much heat in the Lungs, with symptoms such as dry cough that may have specks of blood, with a low-grade fever, and abnormal thirst and sweating.
- *Phlegm in the Lungs (AKA excess mucus)* happens when a person develops phlegm elsewhere in their body, usually from a weak digestive system, and it then develops in the Lungs. In TCM, the Spleen (and the digestive system) is said to be the creator of phlegm while the Lungs are the container, or receptacle of phlegm. Symptoms here include wheezing, cough, or asthma with coughing up of sticky mucus. Phlegm is

often created when a person eats too many foods that are cold, sweet and fattening.

- *Deficient Lung Qi* has symptoms like shortness of breath, fatigue, and a soft, quiet voice. Such people tend to be low energy and get sick often and very easily.

Death and renewal= the cycle of life

Autumn is the time of year that leaves fall from the trees, and crops are harvested, leaving empty fields. It's a time of year with many deaths. Yet, there is much beauty in this process because death is a natural part of the cycle of life. Death eventually leads to life once again. The Lungs in humans are said to "house the corporeal soul", known as the *Po*. It's the most tangible, physical aspect of our soul. The *Po* is believed to die with our physical body. It's our physical reality, the aspect of our life that is purely about tactile (touch) experiences. By protecting our Lungs, we can think of ourselves as maintaining and extending the life of our most basic, "physical" soul.

Take a deep breath, find some happiness, boundaries and closure

Breathing is involuntary, and so basic to life that we'll die within minutes if we don't take in the oxygen provided by the air. But breathing is so much more than just survival. Ever wonder why people sitting in meditation seem so peaceful? That's a complex answer, but it's in part related to their constant focus on the present moment, being consciously aware of their bodies, and paying close attention to their breathing. When was the last time you CONSCIOUSLY took three long, deep breaths? Why don't you do it now? I'll wait... (insert "Jeopardy" theme song here.)

I'm guessing you already feel better after that short break. Why? You just fed your body with *Qing qi*, or the oxygen and energy from the air. The *Qing qi* combines with the nutrients provided by the food you eat (*Gu qi*), to form the energy that eventually feeds the entire body (known as *Zong qi*). That is how foundational breathing is: it is a necessary part of feeding our entire body. Yet most of us ignore the process. So, I encourage you to start paying attention, today! You can build up your Lungs' strength through simple daily breathing routines, and through regular exercise.

Once you are focused on the physical action of breathing, start to look at the emotions that can relate to breathing. How does this work? Many of us are (figuratively) holding our breaths, stuck living in a sad event from our past. You may have had a major loss, such as the death of a loved one, and can't move on. This can lead to a sense of depression, or "stuckness" that seems never-ending. Activities that focus on your breathing can be very helpful in letting you move forward. Meditation is a great example.

Fueling foods for the Lungs: I hope you like soup!
In general, white and light-colored foods benefit the Lungs, so white meats, white mushrooms, radishes, garlic, and onion are helpful in boosting your Lung health and immune system. Think about the chicken soup we turn to when we have a cold: the white meat, onion*, ginger, pale broth, vegetables and maybe a bit of spicy hot sauce. All of these help your body support the Lung tissue and fight off infection.

*Note: using scallion, or green onion (versus white onion) is actually best if you have a cold. But, you actually want to use the *white* part of the plant near the root to help you recover, which coincidentally also follows the guideline of using white foods to treat Lung issues.

Remember that the fall is a time for turning inward, so it's helpful to eat sour foods that help the body "rein it in" and begin to contract in preparation for winter. Foods like vinegar, yogurt, leeks, lemons, limes, grapefruit, and sourdough bread are good examples.

Fall is also the time that illnesses due to dryness are quite common, such as a dry cough. Eating foods that moisten is helpful at this time. Pears (especially when baked with honey!), apples, loquat fruit, nuts, and many dairy and animal products help combat dryness. Don't go overboard though because you don't want to end up creating too much damp in your body!

To stimulate your sense of smell and appetite, saute and bake your foods for longer periods during the autumn season. Cooking foods at a lower heat for a longer time and with less water is also a good plan during that season.

Foods that drain the Lung energy
You ***absolutely*** must take care to understand what particular type of Lung problem you have (dryness, heat, phlegm, or qi deficiency) in order to eat the correct foods. For instance, if you have too much dryness in your lungs (or your body in general), be careful to avoid most aromatic spices and warming foods because they will further dry the body. But these foods can often help if you have too much phlegm in your Lungs. Double check the grocery list at the end of the chapter and match it to your particular symptoms to ensure you're buying foods that work best for you.

A word on dairy products
Most Americans would probably list cheese as a staple food in their diet. And no, I don't blame you! However, if you have poor digestion, and have signs of too much phlegm in your Lungs, dairy products such as milk, yogurt, and cheese will absolutely make these symptoms worse. On the other hand, if you have Lung dryness, especially if your Lungs are weak and not showing any signs of heat, dairy products in moderation

will help soothe and moisten the mucus membranes. When in doubt as to whether dairy products help or aggravate your health, I recommend you first try other types of foods listed in this chapter for increasing the health or your Lungs versus eating dairy. You can also try eliminating dairy entirely from your diet for several weeks to see how you feel.

Lifestyle ideas: *increase immunity, protect yourself, resolve grievances*
- Exercise often, it moves your qi and increases immunity.

If you aren't physically active, your energy doesn't circulate. This decreases Lung capacity and over time will lower your ability to fight off colds. Your bowel movements may also become irregular, and poor intestinal health decreases your immunity. In fact, most of our body's immune defenses live in the intestines! Stretching movements which physically open the chest particularly increase Lung health. Choose movements that help to stretch the muscles around the ribs and upper body.

- Don't smoke! Breathe instead!

You've heard it before, but it's worth repeating: if you smoke cigarettes, you will likely die because of this habit, from diseases like cancer, stroke or heart attack. In the meantime, you can expect to suffer from frequent colds, bronchitis, and emphysema. There are many resources out there to help you quit, including acupuncture!

In contrast to smoking, let's focus on providing loving care for your Lungs. Again, breathing exercises can help improve your Lung function and capacity. Singing, even off-key, is great! Guided meditations where you focus on breathing are also a good option.

- Dry brush your skin

The skin is an important part of the Lung system and your immunity, and it can be nourished by brushing. Rubbing with a cotton towel or scrubbing using a soft brush stimulates the skin, and brings qi and blood to the area. Wearing natural fabrics like cotton allows the skin to breathe freely.

- Pay attention to the air quality in your environment

The air in our homes is often stagnant and can impair Lung health. We tend to get sick in winter partly because the heater dries out our skin and Lungs, and the closed windows keep out fresh air. There are a number of houseplants that help clean the air in your home, including English ivy, Bamboo palm, Peace lily, and Philodendron. Products such as air purifiers also help clean the air. When possible, open your windows to create airflow, although if you have allergies you likely already know to be careful on days when there is a high pollen count. And keeping your house relatively dust-free and tidy not only helps your Lungs, it will also help you bring more clarity to your thinking and emotions. In fact, maintaining a tidy home can be an important step in recovering from grief because clearing your physical space helps clear your mind to make room for healing.

- Resolve grief

Beyond keeping a tidy house, thus fostering a "respect" for our home environment, we need to respect ourselves and others. Do you feel like you really value who you are, and surround yourself with others who willingly provide you with the emotional support you need? Have you deeply explored your values, needs, and past grievances? Have you truly forgiven yourself and your loved ones? Expressing ourselves by, in essence, using our voices can help to heal and open the energy of the Lungs.

Western biomedical perspective

Many white foods have been found to have antibacterial and antiviral properties and thus help fight off illnesses that affect the Lung. Examples include garlic, ginger, and onions, all of which reduce inflammation and fight infections. Turmeric is related to ginger and has many of the same benefits, including anti-cancer properties! Turmeric contains curcumin, a compound that encourages cancer cells to self-destruct. Onions provide vitamin C, vitamin B6, and other critical nutrients, which feed the body and also have anti-cancer properties. Another component in onions is quercetin, a natural antioxidant, and research has shown it helps prevent Lung diseases including cancer.

Several fruits contain compounds that improve Lung health. Pomegranates appear to slow the growth of Lung tumors, perhaps due to the antioxidant ellagic acid. Apples contain flavonoids and vitamins C and E, all of which help the Lungs function at their best. People who eat several apples a week have been shown to have healthier Lungs. Grapefruit contains the flavonoid naringin, which inhibits the activation of a cancer causing enzyme. Grapefruit has been shown to be especially good at cleansing the Lungs after quitting smoking.

Fatty fish and fish oil supplements offer vitamin D, which appears to have a direct link to Lung health. A deficiency of this vitamin leads to a risk of decreased Lung function. Fatty fish is also rich in omega-3 fatty acids, which support the health of the entire body, including the Lungs. These fatty acids also provide some protection against cancer. For vegetarians, walnuts are a plant source of omega-3 fatty acids.

While white and light-colored foods are good in general for Lung health, keep in mind that orange and dark green vegetables tend to be high in beta carotene (Vitamin A), which helps heal mucus membranes, which are the linings of the Lungs. Apricots, carrot, winter squash, pumpkin, broccoli, kale, mustard greens, and blue-green algae supplements are good examples. Green foods' chlorophyll also helps protect the body from viruses and environmental toxins. Cruciferous vegetables like cabbage, cauliflower, broccoli and kale have been shown to halt the progression of Lung cancer and cut the risk of developing Lung cancer.

Berries are rich in antioxidants, which fight off free radicals that may damage Lungs. Acai and blueberry are particularly rich in free radicals, but cranberries, grapes, and strawberries are good for the Lungs, too. Kidney, pinto, black and other beans are also good sources of antioxidants. Beans, seeds, and nuts also contain rich amounts of magnesium, a mineral that contributes to healthy Lung function.

Eating enough fiber also helps ensure the Lungs and Large Intestine stay healthy, as fiber assists in gently cleansing the body and working to prevent cancers. Pectin fiber, found in fresh produce like apples, cherries, and carrots is especially helpful.

Take Away Message
Food- White and light-colored foods support immune function
Lifestyle- Value yourself and your home environment
Emotion- Resolve your grievances and work to move on from the past

Metal/ Lung Seasonal Style Grocery List
For dryness of the Lung:
Soybeans (soy milk, tempeh, tofu)
Spinach
Radish
Seaweed
White and light-colored fungi/ mushrooms
Apple
Pear
Persimmon
Nuts (like almonds, peanut, pine, sesame)
Honey
Milk and other dairy products
Barley
Millet
Animal products, especially white meats (like clam, crab, eggs, mussel, oyster, pork)
Salt

For reducing heat in the Lungs (note: some overlap with foods to reduce dryness because adding fluids tends to cool, too):
Algaes (like Chlorella and Spirulina)
Seaweed
Soy and tofu
Tomato
Apple
Peach
Pear
Watermelon
Milk and other dairy products

For phlegm in the Lungs:
Garlic
Ginger
Fennel
Flaxseed
Horseradish
Seaweed

Aromatic/ pungent foods to support Lung health and immunity in general:
Chilies
Garlic
Ginger
Onions
Foods with fiber to cleanse the Large Intestines (most whole fruits, whole grains, and vegetables)

Chinese herbs:
NOTE: While many Chinese herbs are also foods, it's important to consult with a TCM practitioner before consuming more than a minimal amount of these products, as a professional will provide you with the proper dosages as well as how to prepare them. (The English, Latin and Chinese names are provided to help you shop more easily for them.)

- Loquat fruit (Latin Eriobotryae Folium, Chinese Pi Pa Ye)—for coughing and dryness of the Lungs. Chinese herbalists use the loquat leaf, not fruit, but both are effective.
- Lychee fruit (Latin Lycii Cortex, Chinese Di Gu Pi)—for severe Lung heat and cough. Like loquat, Chinese herbalists use the lychee leaf.
- Dried asparagus (Latin Asparagi Radix, Chinese Tian Men Dong)—for dry cough
- Green onion stem (Latin Allii bulbus, Chinese Cong Bai) —just the white part of the plant's stem is best, and is used right when you first catch a cold, helping the body sweat and thus help clear out the virus. Fresh ginger and garlic are used in TCM in much the same manner.

CHAPTER SIX: THE WATER PHASE

Have you ever visited a frozen lake in the deepest cold of winter? I lived in Minnesota for several years and vividly remember the one (and only) time I was brave enough to walk on the ice of a frozen lake. The temperature outside was brutal and my ears felt frozen. The lake was covered in a thick layer of ice and snow and looked as stable as a trail you'd walk on with some snowshoes. Yet, I was still terrified that I'd fall through. I knew the ice was very stable underneath me, but after looking down at the slow-moving blue water far below, so dark and foreboding, I high-tailed back to the safety of solid ground after only a few minutes. The fear had gotten the best of me and I ran as quickly as I could! This experience sums up the character of the water phase and the subject of this chapter: **the Kidneys, wintertime, the emotion fear and dark blue and black foods.**

The Kidneys' important role in our bodies: Water, water, everywhere!

Water relates to the **Kidneys** and their paired organ the Urinary Bladder. These organs help regulate fluid movement around and out of the body, and in TCM the Kidneys are also closely linked to growth, development and reproduction. In TCM, the Kidneys are also thought to contain the basic genetic material we inherit from our parents and play a major role in the early development of vital organs such as the brain and spinal cord. Thus, having strong Kidneys both before and after birth it is crucial to your overall health throughout your life. In fact, if you develop a chronic disease at some point, one of the best ways TCM practitioners can address your illness is by supporting the Kidneys' energy, because any long-term disease becomes part of the basic structure of your body.

The Kidneys: our body's foundation

The health of the Kidneys is tied to many important body functions, including water metabolism, and they're also the storage place of our *Jing*, or essence energy. The quality of Essence depends on both the health you inherit from your parents and how you live your life (especially your diet). When our *Jing* is strong and healthy, we are vital and have a strong ability to fight off disease and live a long life. Signs of weak *Jing* include impaired growth and development as a child, weak legs and bones, and poor brain function. Other signs relate to our reproductive system: infertility and loss of "vital fluids", including excessive vaginal discharge or premature ejaculation. The adrenal glands are also related to the Kidneys. They respond to stress by secreting hormones like cortisol, as well as helping to balance the hormones, especially the sex hormones.

Common symptoms related to poor Kidney health include:
- ringing in the ears (tinnitus), early deafness or other ear problems
- early graying of the hair or baldness
- low libido or other sexual dysfunction
- feeling cold all the time
- chronic low back and knee pain or any problems with the bones
- swelling (edema) of body tissues, especially in the legs and feet
- chronic urinary problems
- an overall feeling of dryness (the mouth and throat in particular) and sweating for no reason
- an unusual amount of insecurity and fear
- poor memory

Signs of deficiency of the Kidney organ system can often be divided into heat and cold types (known as *Yin* versus *Yang* deficiency.) These are discussed below in the section on foods to fuel Kidney health.

Jump right into the deep end!

People with a Water Seasonal Style can feel easily intimidated and lack the will to follow through because their fears stop them from taking action. For instance, you may be like me and feel terrified of drowning. A good solution to that **fear** would be to face it head on and take some swimming lessons! In fact, I now recognize that the more that I fear something (relating to career, family, home, etc.) and the more I want to avoid it, the more it should be faced directly. Basically, the lesson is to jump into the deep end of the "pool of life". This can be hard, however, if you have a weak Kidney organ system, because that weakness can lead to unfounded fears.

How does an unhealthy level of fear play out in the body? If you have too much fear due to the Kidneys being weak (deficient), think of it as having too much water. We all know water can extinguish a fire. Having an excess of water of the Kidney can actually put out too much your "fire", which relates to your Heart and spirit. With too much water and not enough fire, the normal feelings of joyful expression and love that come from the Heart energy can be pushed aside by an unbalanced number of fears and insecurities.

What can cause our fears to spill over beyond healthy caution? Often, it's due to living an "extreme" lifestyle. Think of it in terms of burning off your healthy *Jing* (essence energy) reserves. Once your "gas tank" of *Jing* is completely empty, you're basically dead! It's possible you inherited a weakness of *Jing* from your parents and you have to work to maintain your "low tank". Or, you can burn out that *Jing* fuel too quickly: if you're constantly working, stressed out, living in the fast lane of life (is it like a music video with sex, drugs, rock & roll?) and you eat too many of the wrong foods, then you're probably draining these reserves too quickly.

Rest and recuperate: "be the bear"

One excellent way to maintain your Kidneys' fuel tanks is to carve out regular, meaningful times to rest your body and mind. We all know that many bears hibernate in the **wintertime.** Why? Their innate intelligence tells them it's time to prepare for the coming year by slowing down, resting (A LOT!), and retreating from the world for awhile by hiding in their caves. Winter in the natural world is a time for rest, like the fallow field waiting for spring's plantings of new crops. Winter is the end of the seasons and a time for healing in preparation for the transition to spring and new life.

You may find yourself mimicking the solitary behavior of the bear in the winter, too, especially if you are a Water Seasonal Style. This is a good thing! Consciously slowing down and relaxing, doing quiet, solitary activities such as reading or cooking at home are good choices during wintertime. Because there are fewer hours of sunlight, we should sleep longer to recuperate from the "go go go" nature of the rest of the year.

A Water/ Kidney person may need this type of "bear-like" activity all year round, and often they are considered an introvert by their loved ones. Regularly pulling back to recuperate from the business of life is a normal, healthy solution for Water Seasonal Style people. If this is your dominant Seasonal Style, you are likely drained by too much social interaction or crowded places, and learning how to identify when you need a break from the hustle and bustle of life can be an important part of self-care.

Fueling foods for the Kidney: *think hot or cold, then black and salty*

If you are a Water Seasonal Style, when you consider any changes to your diet, you must determine whether you have a deficiency in the Kidney *Yin* or *Yang*. If you have a lack of *Kidney Yin*, you will probably have too much heat in your body. This causes symptoms such as irritability and fear, hot flashes, dizziness, ear ringing, dry mouth, low back pain, weak limbs, involuntary seminal emission, and hot hands and feet. On the other hand, if you lack *Kidney Yang*, you will have too much cold in your body. You may have the following symptoms: mental slowness, lack of will power, lethargy, low sex drive, frequent and clear urine, asthma, edema, and either a dislike of coldness and/or a feeling of coldness (especially in your arms and legs).

Once you've determined if you're too hot or too cold, you can then choose foods that truly nourish your Kidneys; see the Grocery list at the end of the chapter for specific foods that nourish Kidney *Yin* versus *Yang*. But to support your Kidneys' health in general, dark blue and black foods are nurturing, especially beans and berries. Seafood and other animal products like cheese and eggs are good choices as well. Grains such as millet, barley, oats, quinoa and amaranth are also great options to build Kidney energy. Last, cook your foods for a longer time and at a lower temperature during the winter season.

Foods that drain the Kidney energy
Much like the list of fueling foods for the Kidneys, this list also depends on whether you have too little Kidney *Yin* or *Yang*. Too many hot foods, especially coffee and alcohol, can put a strain on the Kidney *Yin* and the adrenals. Lamb and certain spices (for example, cinnamon, cloves and ginger) are also quite warm and should be eaten in small amounts if you have Kidney *Yin* deficiency. If you have Kidney *Yang* deficiency, you should avoid eating too many "cold" foods. In TCM, "cold" foods include raw fruits and vegetables, as well as frozen and iced foods like ice cream and soy and dairy products.

Salty foods help root the energy deep inside the body, encouraging that "hunkering down" feeling you need in winter, and some dietary salt is necessary for the body's cells to function to function properly. But in general, too much salt intake actually can be damaging to the Kidneys in the long-term. Keep in mind that what matters most is **how much** salt you're eating **and where** you're getting your salt. For instance, did you know that the daily recommended salt intake is only about one teaspoon? And, are you eating highly-processed foods that contain large amounts of added salt versus adding a very small amount of high quality salt to home cooked meals?

Last, eating a large amount of protein (especially highly processed meats and other animal products) is thought to potentially damage the function of the Kidneys in the long-term. See the section on the Western biomedical perspective for more on this issue.

Lifestyle ideas: *Nourish your precious Jing*
As noted above, the Kidneys store the *Jing*, and once you use all that up, you are done for! You must protect your essence, and people often burn theirs out too early due to the stressors of modern life. Are you overdoing it in some aspect of your life? It's very important to be critical and honest with yourself here!

- Do you work too much? If you're working so much that you don't have adequate time to eat decent meals, rest, or have any fun, you're burning up that essence.
- How's your sex life? Rarely having sex or having it very frequently directly affects the health of the Kidneys. Too much semen loss, especially for older men, strains the Kidneys. For women, multiple abortions, miscarriages, and/or childbirths can place undue strain on the Kidneys because they often lead to significant blood loss.
- Are you exercising too much? Yes, this is actually possible! People that exercise for several hours per day doing intense, draining activities like running or weight lifting often end up with serious Kidney deficiency symptoms such as urinary problems, bone fractures, and sexual dysfunction.

- Are you fighting the natural aging process? We all get old, let's face it—don't take crazy products to try and falsely boost yourself up, because these actually have the opposite effect over time and end up draining your essence. It's fine to eat natural, anti-aging foods in moderation. But be honest with yourself if you're starting to overdo it, as even natural products like Ginseng should be taken in moderation.
- Are you taking strong supplements to boost your athletic or sexual performance? Products such as protein shakes have been "all the rage" lately, but much like anti-aging products, they drain the *Jing* over time, having the opposite effect of what you're intending.

The TCM answer to our hectic lives is simple: find balance. You may need to be creative in order to address where in your life you're overdoing it. Is it possible to work less? Can you take it easy on the exercise marathons? Are you getting proper rest and nutrition? If you have a tendency to really aggressively go after *everything* in your life, it's important to be very honest with yourself about how balanced those behaviors are.

Western biomedical perspective
Much of the published information linking diet and nutrition to Kidney health relates to people who already have Kidney disease. Such people most often need to follow a special diet that limits their intake of protein, salt, and fluids, and emphasizes the balance of vitamins and minerals in the body. The research appears controversial and somewhat preliminary regarding how diet could potentially affect the *prevention* of Kidney disease. As an example, too much animal protein in the diet is bad if you already have Kidney disease. Protein is required to create and repair cells, and it is present in every one of our body's cells. Sources of protein include dairy, meat, fish, beans, and grains. But, based on the available research, it can be difficult to say in the long run that you will develop Kidney

disease from excessive protein intake. As with anything, moderation makes the most sense.

The adrenal glands are associated with the Kidneys, and much like the Kidneys, their functioning is affected by overdoing it. If you're stressed, your body pumps out more stress hormones, and if this continues for a long period of time, the adrenals won't work as well. To keep the adrenals healthy, you need to focus on three issues: regular mealtimes, avoiding foods that give you a quick energy boost, and managing stress. Eating at regular times during the day, and eating most of your food earlier in the day, helps maintain your blood sugar and cortisol levels. In addition, it's common to reach for foods such as sugar and caffeine—which give an instant energy boost—if you have adrenal fatigue and stress. Unfortunately, such foods backfire because they will eventually drain the adrenals even more. Last, managing stress helps keep the adrenals from constantly pumping out those stress hormones, which over time lessens the glands' ability to properly function.

Take Away Message

Food- Dark blue and black foods, and a small but healthy amount of salt
Lifestyle- Rest, recover and retreat into your cave to nourish your *Jing*
Emotion- A bit of fear is healthy, too much will paralyze you

Water/ Kidney Seasonal Style Grocery List

Dark blue/ black foods:
Beans (black, kidney)
Black sesame seeds
Blackberry
Blueberry
Mullberry
Spirulina
Chlorella

Foods to nourish Kidney Yin:
Beans (most types, see above)
Berries (see above)
Watermelon and other melons
Grains (barley, millet)
Nuts (chestnuts, walnuts)
Seeds (black sesame, flax, pumpkin, sunflower)
Animal products (cheese, duck, eggs, pork, soups with bone marrow)
Seafoods (clam, crab, sardine)

Foods to nourish Kidney Yang:
Black beans
Onions (including anise, chive, fennel, leeks and scallions)
Walnuts
Quinoa
Meats (chicken, lamb)
Seafood (salmon, trout)
Warming spices (black pepper, cinnamon, cloves, ginger)

Foods with healthier sources of salt:
Seaweed
Miso
Seafoods (sardine, crab, clam)

Chinese herbs:

NOTE: While many Chinese herbs are also foods, it's important to consult with a TCM practitioner before consuming more than a minimal amount of these products. A professional will advise you on proper dosage and preparation. (The English, Latin and Chinese names are provided to help you shop more easily for them.)

- Walnut (Latin Juglandis Semen, Chinese Hu Tao Ren) —nourishes Kidney Yang
- Dried asparagus (Latin Asparagi Radix, Chinese Tian Men Dong—nourishes Kidney Yin and generates fluids

CHAPTER SEVEN: THE WOOD PHASE

Don't you love spring? Each time you go outside, there's a new tree blooming, or a colorful flower bursting forth from the soil. It's a feeling of activity, an "up and out" sensation, where the life in the plant can't help but emerge into the world and show off its beauty. Everything looks so green, abundant and full of life... And as you walk outside, you may notice the wind blowing on your skin. The wind may make you feel a bit irritable and pushed around, but you remind yourself the wind is really a gift because it helps to pollinate all those growing plants. This sums up the character of the wood phase and the subject of this chapter: *the Liver, springtime, the emotion anger and green foods.*

The Liver's important role in our bodies: Move that *Qi*!

Wood relates to the Liver and its paired organ the Gallbladder. According to TCM, the Liver keeps the energy of the body flowing properly, controls the tendons and ligaments, and stores blood. The Liver also is said to "house the soul", which I'll discuss later in the chapter. The Gallbladder stores and excretes bile to aid in the digestion of our food, and it also helps us maintain our emotions and make decisions.

People with Wood Seasonal Styles commonly have health symptoms that relate to their *Qi* (energy) moving too slowly and inefficiently around the body. Common symptoms related to lack of *Qi* movement in the body include: problems with the tendons and ligaments; swellings or lumps around the body (whether benign or cancerous); mild depression; visual disorders like cataracts, glaucoma, or itchy, red eyes; and "wind" disorders like epilepsy, migraines, itchy skin, and dizziness. Stuck Liver *Qi* tends to make people overly irritable, angry, and impatient.

And because the Liver stores the blood, women with a Wood Seasonal Style often have menstrual issues such as tender breasts, PMS, and growths such as uterine fibroids and ovarian cysts.

When people have a Liver imbalance over a long period of time, they also tend to develop signs indicating they have too much heat in their bodies. These symptoms include: constipation, avoiding hot weather, wanting to drink very cold fluids, red and inflamed eyes, migraine headache on the temples or very top of the head, high blood pressure, and extreme, angry outbursts.

Wow, it's so windy outside. All that crazy energy—don't go all Green Hulk!
How do the flowers pollinate in the spring? (Well, besides the hard work of the bees.) The winds of *springtime* are a crucial part of all the new growth, helping pollen float from plant to plant. All that outward movement and growth and windy weather during spring is great, but it can lead to a sense of frenetic, impatient energy inside our bodies. People tend to have an emotional response to this type of weather; they may feel angry, irritable and short tempered.

Remember the comic book called the Green Hulk? The main character, Bruce Banner, seemed like a normal man until he became upset and angry. When that happened, his body would grow in size so much that he'd bust apart his clothes, his skin turned green, and then he'd practically scare everyone to death because he was so angry! If you're a Wood Seasonal Style, you probably know how Bruce felt. It can be a challenge to stop your crabby outbursts when you're this type of Seasonal Style. Thankfully, there are changes you can make to your lifestyle and food choices to help soothe your Liver and chill out all those crabby emotions!

Fueling foods for the Liver: Think sweet-natured Popeye, not the Green Hulk!

In spring we often naturally eat less and eat lighter foods (versus heavy, rich foods), especially those that are "new growth" like fresh greens, and sweet, starchy vegetables and grains. These light foods are often green in color, too. Looking for *green foods* while at the grocery stores is a simple tip to remember when you want to nourish your Liver. If you nourish your Liver with green foods, and other foods like those listed in the Grocery List at the end of the chapter, you can become more like the sweet-natured comic book character Popeye, who as you may remember, always ate his spinach!

Shopping tip: remember when shopping at this time of year and/or for the Wood Seasonal Style to picture a spring garden with lots of new plants bursting forth.

Starchy vegetables like carrots and beets, as well as grains, beans and seeds provide a wonderful flavor to dishes. Seasoning your foods with pungent herbs such as basil is a great choice as well this time of year because the nature of many fresh herbs is light and lifting, like a plant growing up and out.

Raw foods are a great choice, especially if you tend to have a lot of heat in your body. (Be careful to not overdo your serving sizes though, since eating too many raw foods puts a strain on our digestive organs!) Examples of raw foods include fresh fruits and vegetables, beans, seeds, and sprouted grains. And when you do cook your food, cook it quickly and at high heat. Sauteed vegetables are great in springtime!

Foods that drain the Liver energy

Many of the problems related to the Liver are caused by poor movement of the *Qi*, and this is commonly a result of overeating, so one very important step to take to improve the health of your Liver can be to eat less overall, or to eat more often but less food at each meal. Poor movement of the body's Qi is also caused by eating too many fats, heavy foods, and pro-cessed foods. Avoiding foods like meats, fried foods, cheese, eggs, and alcohol, as well as those foods with excess salt (soy sauce, cured meats, etc.) is a helpful habit when you're trying to cleanse your Liver's energetic system.

Lifestyle ideas: *Angry much?*
As mentioned above, all the outward movement and growth during spring is great for the new plants and flowers, but it can lead to that sudden Green Hulk feeling where you're irritable and annoyed at just about anyone and everything near you. There are several simple techniques to help you decompress from crabby moods so that you "survive" the season, and move away from those uncomfortable and irritable feelings that may be present all year:

- Schedule time to laugh in your calendar! Watch some comedy DVDs, search out your funny friends, or read a light-hearted book.
- Calm down... exercises like yoga or Tai Chi help move the body's energy and also help you leave behind any worries of the day.
- Rise early in the day and take a fast-paced walk to get your energy moving. This helps you start your day out more smoothly and assist the Liver in moving your en-ergy.
- Be present in the moment. Simply acknowledge and be conscious that, WOW, it is indeed spring and that things are going to be kind of chaotic in nature. Go one step further by taking breathers to laugh at your (and others') grumbling behavior.
- Watch out for windy, dry weather. That type of weather greatly affects the Liver's energetic system and will of-ten aggravate your symptoms. Cover up in weather like this with a jacket and scarf.
- Avoid relying on sleeping pills or other drugs whenever possible, as they put stress on the Liver and can even-tually cause deficiency of the organ.

Western biomedical perspective

Leafy greens like spinach and lettuce have the ability to neutralize metals, chemicals and pesticides that may be in our foods, and since the Liver is the primary organ for filtering toxins in our bodies, eating greens can boost Liver health. Eating avocados can help your body produce a type of antioxidant called glutathione, which is required for the Liver to filter out harmful materials. (Walnuts also contain glutathione.) Cruciferous veggies like broccoli and brussel sprouts help improve enzyme production that assists in digestion. Garlic helps your Liver activate the enzymes that can flush out toxins. Grapefruit and its juice can help your Liver flush out toxins and the fruit is also high in both vitamin C and antioxidants. Green tea contains antioxidants known as catechins, which have been known to improve the function of our Liver. For the Gallbladder, the spice turmeric helps to digest fats and stimulate the production of bile.

Take Away Message

Food- Green foods, raw foods, and new growth plants like a springtime garden
Lifestyle- The active time of year, take advantage of the abundant, new energy
Emotion- Be physically active, but make sure to mentally chill out: take a deep breath because anger hurts you, not them

Wood/ Liver Seasonal Style Grocery List
Green foods:
Asparagus
Broccoli
Brussel sprouts
Greens (chard, collard, kale, kohlrabi, mustard)
Kelp
Lettuce (Romaine)
Parsley
Seaweed
Spinach
Chlorophyll-rich foods (Blue-green algae, Spirulina, Wheat grass)

Foods to help *Qi* move more smoothly:
Grains
Legumes
Natural sweeteners (honey, molasses, whole cane sugar)
Vinegar (apple cider or any other unrefined and organic vinegar)
Citrus (lemon, lime or grapefruit)

Other herbs and foods that improve Liver health:
Basil
Bay leaf
Cardamom
Dill
Fennel
Rosemary
Cherries
Strawberries
Peaches
Onions (all types)
Mushrooms
Radish
Rhubarb
Starchy vegetables (beets, carrots, etc.)
Liver organ meat

Chinese herbs:

NOTE: While many Chinese herbs are also foods, it's important to consult with a TCM practitioner before consuming more than a minimal amount of these products, as a professional will provide you with the proper dosages as well as how to prepare them. (The English, Latin and Chinese names are provided to help you shop more easily for them.)

- Jujube seed (Latin Ziziphi Spinosae Semen, Chinese Suan Zao Ren)—nourishes Liver blood
- Sour moutain date (Latin Corni Fructus, Chinese Shan Zhu Yu)—nourishes Liver and Kidney
- Peony root (Latin Peony radix, Chinese Bai Shao)—for many Liver issues
- Dandelion root (Latin Taraxacum officinalis, Chinese Pu Gong Ying)—for severe Liver heat, for painful urination, eye problems, mastitis and abscess

CHAPTER EIGHT: EXCESS WEIGHT and TCM

Let me begin this chapter by first stating that we fixate entirely too much on how much we *weigh* versus how good we actually *feel*. If more of us would focus instead on our well-being versus what the bathroom scale says, we'd be so much better off. (This idea is discussed in more detail later in this chapter in the section on emotions.) I encourage you to always keep this thought in the back of your mind, especially when you're having a really self-critical moment. Turning the blame back on yourself rarely leads to healthy progress!

Throughout this chapter, I will use the term "excess weight" and never talk about "weight loss". There is too much emphasis placed on the idea of losing weight. The weight loss industry, full of fad diets and supplements, banks on this emphasis. You absolutely may want to lose that weight and never find it again! But, let's start from reality, and with no judgment, just fact: most of us have some excess weight on our body frames.

There are many reasons we as a society have collectively gained so much excess weight in the past few generations; however, that discussion is beyond the scope of this book. What I do want to point out is that many of the supposed "causes" of our high rates of obesity have been aimed at blaming the individual. We've been told that we are weak, horrible failures. But there are many societal and biological factors, too, unrelated to whether we have enough willpower to resist eating JUST ONE MORE candy bar. What about the quality of our food, or lack thereof? What about the presence of pollutants in the environment, which not only cause illness, but disrupt our hormones, leading to weight gain? There are many prescription drugs that cause weight gain. And in many areas of the U.S., access to affordable, fresh, local, and organic foods is very limited. This is such a complex challenge and the questions and reasons for obesity go on and on. I do talk about a couple of these issues here in this chapter, but most of the causes of obesity are way beyond what we can cover here. I encourage you to educate yourself about the issue!

In this chapter, we'll focus our attention on five topics:
- The TCM theories that explain excess weight
- Issues you may not have considered that relate to your eating habits and meal times
- Why movement is important but not the "be-all and end-all"
- The role that emotions play in your diet
- Other medical issues that may be factors.

You'll notice that in this chapter the writing is in contrast to many medical weight loss programs and products, which tend to *ONLY focus on controlling hunger and cravings—NOT the other common factors contributing to excess weight.* **And why then do most dieters gain the weight back? Because they've used a band aid approach. They haven't solved the underlying issues.**

Topic one: TCM theories on excess weight
It may shock you to hear a health care provider say that excess weight is often caused by your body not working as well as it should, rather than just talking about your food choices or other behavior. (Bad dieter!!) But that is exactly what the knowledge provided by TCM theories points to: if someone is overweight or obese, it's likely due to a dysfunction or disharmony inside their body. And, yes, diet and behavior commonly lead to such disharmonies, but they aren't the only causes. TCM above all is about restoring and maintaining balance. Fat in the body is necessary and desirable—you don't want too little or too much. Having either an overweight (*fei pang*) or too thin (*xiao shou*) body type is undesirable.

There are three organ systems in the body related to excess weight: the Spleen/ Stomach, the Liver, and the Kidneys. (If you haven't read the earlier chapters in this book on the Earth, Wood, and Water Seasonal Styles, I encourage you to do so. They list more specific details than are given here.)

First and most important is the **Spleen/ Stomach**. A weak digestive system is probably the most common dysfunction in Western societies that leads to weight gain. (Please note that here we also include the function of the pancreas, which plays a significant role in digestion, particularly the metabolism of sugars.) An excess of fat in the body is considered by TCM to be an accumulation of unhealthy "stuck" fluids, which congeal and cause excess mucus, which then produce excess fat. This excess is usually caused by a weakened Spleen, which is in charge of changing our food into useful nutrients and fluids.

Eating too many of the wrong foods is often what causes the Spleen to function poorly and become weak. A helpful tip here is to not eat too many COLD and SWEET foods. Examples of cold foods are: foods like ice cream and iced tea that are literally cold in temperature, as well as other foods that have a cooling effect on the body (which include raw, uncooked vegetables and fruits, and soy and dairy products). Examples of sweet foods are: cookies and other desserts, pastas and breads, sweeteners like honey and maple syrup, and foods (especially fruits) that are naturally high in sugar like dates. In addition, consuming too many fatty and greasy foods, and overeating in general also weaken our Spleen.

Frequently, a patient comes to see me and is confused: she's eating a healthy green salad and a blended fruit smoothie every day, but her weight hasn't budged. Sadly, she has sabotaged her efforts because her digestive system is overwhelmed, cold and working too hard!

There are other reasons the Spleen/ Stomach can become weak. If you don't exercise enough hours during the week, if you constantly work and/or worry about an important aspect of your life, or if you have any other chronic stressors, you most likely have a somewhat weak digestive system. Digestive problems such as loose stools or constipation, fatigue with a heavy feeling in the arms and legs, gas and bloating, and acid reflux are common signs that occur with a weakened digestive system.

Closely tied to the health of the digestive organs is the health of *the Liver's energy*. The Liver is the second organ system related to excess weight. If you have too much stress and don't handle your emotions in a healthy way, the Liver is significantly affected. When the Liver is weakened, it bullies other organ systems to get the nourishment it's lacking. This creates a vicious circle, with a weak Liver leading to a malfunctioning digestive system. It also affects the movement of *qi* (energy, fluids, nutrients, etc.) in the body, and when the *qi* doesn't move properly, nothing else does, either. This is a big factor in the buildup of mucus and dampness in the body, and that buildup leads to weight gain. How does the Liver malfunction? You may know that many medications put a strain on the Liver, but your state of mind can also affect its energy. Feelings of anger, rage, and unfulfilled desires weaken the Liver. And because the Liver in TCM stores the blood, anything that leads to significant blood loss can lead to a weakened Liver. Menstruation, surgery and childbirth are common examples.

The *Kidneys* are the third major organ system that can lead to excess weight. The Kidneys are in charge of the body's fluid metabolism, chiefly the making of urine. And, if the Spleen is weak, it's almost guaranteed that over time, the Kidneys will become weak. As we age, the vitality of the Kidneys naturally decreases. This decline is hastened by things like: an "extreme" lifestyle of overwork and too much or too strenuous physical activity; an enduring, chronic disease; and an overuse of drugs and medications. Also, if a person takes in very large amounts of water, salt and animal protein, this can put a strain on the Kidneys over time. If the Kidneys are weak, it often leads to excess weight due to edema, or too much fluid in the body's tissues.

How are these theories about our organs important? They can help you remember that the internal workings of your body—not just what you put in your mouth or how many hours you log on the Stairmaster—are an important part of weight management. Eating right for your Seasonal Style is of course important, but seeking out a trained health care provider when you need more advice and treatment is crucial: healing your body may take more than just changing your weekly grocery list. Traditional Chinese Medicine, especially when acupuncture and herbal medicine are used in conjunction with dietary changes, is an effective way to restore the health of your organs. Know that it IS possible to make strides—you may just need a different strategy! Don't give up, and seek the advice of a professional!

Topic two: Eating
Most of us have heard the saying "eat less and exercise more." It's a perfect argument to support the bloated diet industry, because if you're not losing weight, obviously you're doing one of those two things wrong! This is a reductive, simplistic view of how our bodies work. I'm hoping that some of the ideas presented here will instead provide you with more tangible, realistic and helpful tools.

Let's now discuss **cooking your food**—at home, on the stove. (It's that metal thing next to the fridge.) Yes, I know, we all work a million hours and have so many other obligations. And sometimes the idea of chopping up a bunch of vegetables seems like an impossible task. But let's be real: cutting up those veggies will probably take you less than five minutes, likely less time than it would take to wait at the drive-in.

One of the most important take-aways for you in this entire book is this: you absolutely must make choosing and cooking healthy foods a serious priority in your life. And I PROMISE that if you actually do make it a priority, your life will change for the better, and in surprising ways that you likely never hoped for—much less expected. But what if you're not sure *how* to cook, *what* to cook, or don't feel in- spired? There are many easy-to-read websites, books, class- es and other resources out there to make cooking fun, fast and easy. Go for it!!

Now let's discuss **conscious eating**. Many people are un- aware that the way they eat, as well as their food choices, can harm their health. Here are *two common and unfortunate scenarios*: in the first, you're late for a work-related lunch meeting, so you stop at a fast food place and absent-mindedly eat while you drive. In the second scenario, you're at home watching TV with your family, arguing with your child, typing on your laptop, and munching on some chips, all at the same time.

What are some of the problems with these two scenarios?
- Lack of focus and attention on the food being eaten
- Multi-tasking with other unrelated activities
- Eating as quickly as possible (shoveling it in!)
- Substituting quick, convenient, packaged and pro- cessed foods for quality home-cooked meals
- Eating while stressed and emotional

Here's *a more optimal, balanced meal time scenario*:
- Set the table, using your best plates, napkins, and dec- orations. Make it a beautiful and serene setting.
- Invite your loved ones to join you for the meal. Set aside any arguments or stressful topics for later. Turn off the TV, and ban cell phones and anything with a video screen from the table.
- Focus only on the meal itself. Really *examine* your plate, appreciate its nutritional value and be grateful for its bounty—it is keeping you alive, after all! You may

even choose to remain silent during the meal to keep you focused on the food.

- Chew each bite of food about 30 times. This saves wear and tear on your digestive organs. (Did you know that an enzyme in our saliva helps to digest carbohydrates?)
- Chewing well also helps you eat more slowly so that your brain realizes what's happening, sees you're getting full, and thus you're less likely to overeat. Putting your fork down after each bite also helps you slow down the pace. A good rule of thumb is to eat until you're not quite full.

Yes, yes I know... every meal you eat isn't going to be this balanced, unhurried and relaxed. But I've listed these details because it is important to be aware that the environment around us while we eat is *extremely* important, and this is an often-overlooked detail in our everyday lives.

Now let's talk about **some options for what foods to eat to maintain a healthy weight**. These foods help provide the nutrition your body requires, heal your digestive system, get your metabolism up and running again, and reduce excess water and damp in the body. Please note that this is by no means a complete list. You must also take care to adapt menus to your own unique health needs, as well as to adjust for any food allergies or food sensitivities.

Fruits: kiwi, mango, papaya, pear, red apples, red grapes, strawberries, watermelon

Vegetables: baby corn, bamboo shoots, broccoli, carrots, cauliflower, celery, eggplant, fennel, green pepper, lotus, mushrooms, onion, tomatoes, scallion, seaweed, squash, zucchini

Nuts, oils and seeds: cashew, coconut, chestnut, olive, pine, safflower, sesame, walnut

Cooking herbs and spices: black and white pepper, chili peppers, cinnamon, clove, garlic, mint

Other foods: unprocessed and local bee pollen and honey, rice, herbal teas

However, I want to emphasize that the **quality of the foods you eat is just as important as what you eat** (colors, types, number of calories/ fats/ carbs, etc.). While this book focuses on the traits of specific foods for each Seasonal Style, it is far better for you to eat **local, organic, whole foods** versus strictly adhere to any one type of food plan, including the one provided in this book. I have the luxury of living in California, where much of the fresh produce supplied to the U.S. is grown. Finding fresh, affordable foods is a big challenge in many places, but do the best you can.

One last aspect to consider for eating and meal times that is rarely discussed is the **differing methods of preparing foods**. It's best to steam or stir-fry your food when possible because these cooking methods only lightly cook the food. This preserves the nutrients and also makes the food relatively easy to digest. You can also stew, boil or bake most of your food if you have a "cold" health condition and need to warm up your digestion. (It's important to remember that eating too many cold and raw foods can negate efforts to lose excess weight because a diet full of cold food hampers the function of the digestive organs.)

Topic three: Movement
No pain, no gain!! Well, sorry, but I have to disagree. I believe that we long ago lost the understanding of *why* physical movement is important, probably sometime during the last century. During the 1900s, and especially with advances in technology, our society shifted from most jobs being labor-intensive and physically demanding to office work where most workers sat all day. Out of necessity, people began "exercis-

ing", whereas before the 20th century that concept was mostly unknown. Exercise, in a sense, replaced the physical hardships of daily life. And research is beginning to show that we may be approaching exercise all wrong—killing yourself at the gym for two hours a couple times each week isn't making up for sitting all day long in your cubicle and then later at home on the couch.

Another way to think about your health and fitness is to focus on the idea of movement. I encourage you to choose exercises that **move your energy**, versus working you so hard your body is strained to the point of exhaustion. Think of your body as an electrical circuit, much like the one in your house. Your energy flows through "wires" (known as *qi meridians* in TCM). Activities such as walking, yoga, martial arts and tai chi help to open the meridians. If you work to open the meridians and keep the energy flowing properly, your health will improve. Of course, getting your heart pumping is obviously important, but this other aspect of movement is just as necessary. Don't worry about logging intense hours at the gym; instead, try to introduce short periods of movement throughout your day. So get out there today, take a walk and do some stretches!

Topic four: Emotions
If you are overweight, chances are you have been personally attacked for how you look, and you certainly have noticed how overweight people are portrayed in our culture. Our society is seriously MEAN to overweight people, even though more than half of all U.S. adults are considered too heavy!!

Above all, be good to yourself. Love yourself and who you are as a person. "Self-love" is still thought of as a dirty word in our culture, and the concept is often compared to being a narcissist. Not true! If you love yourself, you can better understand the role that food has played in your life: it's not supposed to be a crutch to help you cope with your emotions, it is your fuel. Enjoy your food, learn to have a positive relationship with your food, and use your "gut feeling" by paying attention to what your body wants. Your gut will tell you the truth if you listen, and perhaps help you lose the negative baggage about eating that you have accumulated. If you adopt many of the ideas presented in this book, your body will likely tell you more often when to stop eating, and it will begin to have more healthy food desires, rather than cravings for, as an example, processed sugar or deep fried anything.

One helpful activity to try in order to understand your emotional relationship to your weight is **keeping a food journal**. You may have heard that writing down what you eat helps you figure out your diet "blind spots". Tracking how much and what you eat is often quite eye-opening (whoops, I forgot about the three candy bars I ate this week!). A good food journal should not only list what you eat. It should also include 1) what times of the day you're eating, 2) what activities are going on around you that led you to eat, and 3) how you're feeling at that moment (what's motivating you to eat). You can also track any food cravings and any foods you're choosing NOT to eat. Do you see the difference in this type of journal versus obsessively tracking calories, or weighing the exact ounces? Creating a well-rounded food journal will help get to the root of what may seem like insignificant details, but in the long run can identify important, and self-sabotaging food choices.

Topic five: Other medical considerations
Perhaps you've struggled for years with being overweight, tried many diets and products, but your weight doesn't seem to budge. It's a good idea to see a healthcare professional and perhaps have some lab tests, especially if you have had difficulty losing weight for a long time, or you've had a significant weight change in a short period of time.

Often, people struggling to lose weight have **an underlying, unidentified health issue that contributes to their excess weight**. Here are three common examples:

- Millions of people have an undiagnosed thyroid disorder that causes their metabolism to be sluggish; often, these people cannot lose weight no matter how hard they try.
- Many others have stressed adrenal glands, leading to an unbalanced level of the cortisol hormone, which easily leads to weight gain, especially around the abdominal area.
- Last, a large percentage of people have sensitivities or allergies to certain foods that they may not be aware of, which can lead as well to excess weight because the digestive system doesn't function at its best.

There are very effective blood and saliva tests that can easily and definitively diagnose thyroid diseases, hormone imbalances, food allergies, and many other significant health problems. Let me stress here the importance of finding a progressive doctor—doctors using "functional medicine", which includes comprehensive lab work are a great example. Naturopaths, Osteopaths, and Licensed Acupuncturists are great resources, as are many Medical Doctors.

Another often overlooked cause of excess weight is prescription medication. Some examples of prescription medications that have been associated with weight gain include: antidepressants such as TCAs and SSRIs (Paxil, Prozac, Remeron, Vanatrip), anticonvulsants/ mood stabilizers (Depakote, Lithium, Neurontin), antihistamines (Allegra, Zyrtec), antipsychotics (Clozaril, Thorazine, Zyprexa), diabetes medications (DiaBeta, Glucotrol), anithypertensive beta blockers (Lopressor, Tenormin), oral corticosteroids (Deltasone, prednisone), and the progestin-only injectable birth control called depomedroxyprogesterone acetate (DMPA). If you are taking one of these medications, DO NOT stop on your own. This can be very dangerous. Consult your doctor about any concerns instead.

A check-up and consultation with your doctor is always a good idea if you're making any significant diet or lifestyle change.

Getting a proper lab workup can provide you with a "baseline" to start from as you work to improve your overall health, and you could also discuss with them any prescription drugs that may be affecting your weight.

Taking it all in
This chapter has covered five areas related to excess weight: the TCM theories related to digestion, tips on healthier eating and meal times, a new way of looking at exercise, the role of emotions, and some underlying medical issues that may be factors. Hopefully it is now very clear that counting calories and logging countless hours at the gym make up only one small part of your journey towards better health and a more optimal body weight.

CHAPTER NINE: Some Concluding Thoughts

I'll happily state this again: my purpose for writing this book has been to help you learn a new way of thinking about your health, your body, and how to be more connected to nature and the seasons. One way to do that is by identifying what dominant Seasonal Style resonates with you, and thus what foods will best fuel the unique needs of your body.

Traditional Chinese Medicine, especially the Five Phase theory, suggests that people are typically born with a body type that mirrors one the five seasons of the year. And as a result, each person tends to have nutritional needs, health challenges, and a personality type that correspond to "their" season. What I hope is now abundantly clear to you is that these theories are so powerful precisely because you can use them to improve your health organically, in a natural way.

Here is a summary of the main take away points provided in each of the five Seasonal Style chapters:

FIRE/ HEART/ SUMMER
Food- Red colors, full of fluid, with cooling properties
Lifestyle- Be active and engaged but take time to quiet your mind
Emotion- Do what makes you feel joyful and spend time with happy people

EARTH/ SPLEEN/ EARLY FALL
Food- Yellow and orange colored, hearty rice porridges, but limit the damp foods
Lifestyle- Create a regular schedule but stay flexible so you can adjust to change
Emotion- Don't let yourself fall into those pensive, worrisome thoughts—take action instead

METAL/ LUNG/ LATE FALL
Food- White and light-colored foods support immune function
Lifestyle- Value yourself and your home environment
Emotion- Resolve your grievances and work to move on from the past

WATER/ KIDNEYS/ WINTER
Food- Dark blue and black foods rule the Kidneys, as does a small but healthy amount of salt
Lifestyle- Rest, recover and retreat into your cave to nourish your *Jing*
Emotion- A bit of fear is healthy, too much will paralyze you

WOOD/ LIVER/ SPRING
Food- Green foods, raw foods, and new growth plants like those found in a springtime garden
Lifestyle- It's an active time of year, take advantage of the abundant energy
Emotion- Be physically active, but make sure to mentally chill out: take a deep breath because anger hurts you, not them

Thank you for reading *Food for the Five Seasons*! You should now be able to:
- Identify the signs and symptoms that show how you may be out of balance with your natural Seasonal Style
- Empower yourself to take charge of your own health by making simple food choices and adjustments to your daily living
- Reduce your chronic health struggles (pain, sleeping problems, poor digestion, anxiety and depression, etc...)
- Reinvent your grocery list

I sincerely hope that you now adopt the knowledge provided by these ancient, amazing and time-tested theories. If you do so, I believe that you will truly improve your health and well-being, all while living harmoniously with nature and the passing seasons.

CHAPTER TEN: Some Book Resources

As I mentioned in the introduction, there aren't many easy-to-read and accessible books about Traditional Chinese Medicine where a lay person can learn to apply these ancient ideas in their own life. However, there are a few wonderful resources out there that go into much more detail than this book, especially as they relate to using TCM nutritional advice for addressing excess weight. Here are several books that I recommend for those seeking more advice and information:

Ancient Wisdom, Modern Kitchen: Recipes from the East for Health, Healing and Long Life. Yuan Wang, Warren Sheir and Mika Ono. Cambridge, MA: Da Capo Press, 2010.

Chinese Medicine & Health Weight Management: An Evidence-Based Approach. Juliette Aiyana, L.Ac. Boulder, CO: Blue Poppy Press, 2007.

Healing with Whole Foods: Asian Traditions and Modern Nutrition, Third edition. Paul Pitchford. Berkeley, CA: North Atlantic Books, 2002.

Real Food All Year: Eating Seasonal Whole Foods for Optimal Health and All-Day Energy. Nishanga Bliss, MSTCM, L.Ac. Oakland, CA: New Harbinger Publications, 2012.

The Tao of Healthy Eating: Dietary Wisdom According to Chinese Medicine, Second edition. Bob Flaws. Boulder, CO: Blue Poppy Press, 2010.

The Tao of Nutrition, 3rd ed. Maoshing Ni, Ph.D., O.M.D. and Cathy McNease, B.S., Dipl.C.H. Los Angeles, CA: Tao of Wellness Press, 2009.

Traditional Chinese Medicine: A Natural Guide to Weight Loss that Lasts. Nan Lu, O.M.D., M.S. L.Ac. and Ellen Schaplowsky. New York, NY: HarperCollins, 2000.

APPENDIX 1: *Seasonal Style Symptom Indicator*

1) It will take you approximately 20 minutes to complete this indicator checklist.

2) Place a check mark beside any symptoms below that you currently have, or have had in the past. Some items relate to your emotions and your habits, not just health concerns. Some items aren't necessarily symptoms of a health problem, but they do relate to a particular Seasonal Style.

3) Add up the number of items you checked under each of the five categories. The category with the most check marks is your dominant Seasonal Style.

4) You may fall into more than one Seasonal Style. For instance, you may check nine symptoms for Wood, five symptoms for Earth, and three symptoms for Water. That means you are predominantly a Wood Seasonal Style, but could likely benefit from learning about the Earth and Water Seasonal Styles as well.

5) This is not an exhaustive list. See a professional healthcare provider if you have further questions or need guidance. This list is not intended as medical advice or treatment.

6) Note: there are "normal" or balanced attributes that relate to each Seasonal Style. The inventory looks instead mostly at the imbalances in your health that relate to your dominant Seasonal Style.

FIRE/ HEART/ SUMMER

☐High or low blood pressure	☐Easily startled or panicked
☐Cardiovascular disease	☐Often anxious
☐Prescribed a blood thinner medication (Warfarin)	☐Laugh very loudly
☐Stroke (CVA or TIA)	☐Talk almost incessantly
☐Pacemaker	☐Speech problems (stuttering, aphasia)
☐Racing heart/ palpitations	☐Tongue ulcers/ sores
☐Chest/ angina pain	☐Night sweats
☐Hyperthyroidism	☐Insomnia, especially restless sleep
☐Varicose veins	☐Nightmares and/or many vivid dreams

EARTH/ SPLEEN/ EARLY FALL

☐Bruise Easily	☐Diabetes
☐Diarrhea	☐Overweight
☐Constipation	☐Hemorrhoids
☐Digestive disorder (Colitis, Crohns, Diverticulitis, IBS, etc.)	☐Prolapse (stomach, uterus, rectum)
☐Frequent nausea	☐Crave/ often eat greasy, fatty foods
☐Heartburn/ acid reflux	☐Crave/ often eat cold foods and/or dairy foods
☐Low appetite	☐Crave/ often eat sweet foods
☐Frequent hunger	☐Recent antibiotic use
☐Bad breath	☐Frequently worry about life, which can prevent you from falling asleep at night
☐Fatigue	
☐Weak, heavy arms and legs	
☐Muscle wasting/ atrophy	☐Depression, apathy

METAL/ LUNG/ LATE FALL

☐Skin disease (rash, Eczema, Psoriasis) ☐Frequent colds and flus ☐Swollen lymph glands ☐Seasonal allergies/ Food sensitivities ☐Asthma ☐Smoke cigarettes ☐Hoarse voice ☐Rarely sweat, or sweat frequently ☐Dry, brittle body hair ☐Significant amount of body hair	☐Sinus/ nasal problems (stuffy, sneezing, loss of sense of smell, nose bleed) ☐Bronchitis ☐Chronic lung disease (emphysema, COPD) ☐Tuberculosis ☐Grieving from a loss (even from long ago) ☐Frequent weeping ☐ Chronic cough ☐Shortness of breath

WATER/ KIDNEY/ WINTER

☐Birth defect/ developmental delay

☐Low back pain

☐Knee problems

☐Arthritis/ bursitis/ tendonitis

☐Ruptured/ bulging vertebrae

☐Osteoporosis/ brittle, broken bones

☐Urinary disorders (painful urination, incontinence, blood in urine)

☐Kidney Stones

☐Frequent urination, especially at night

☐Poor determination/ will power

☐Decreased short-term memory

☐Hearing impairment/ deafness

☐Tinnitus/ ear ringing

☐Serious chronic disease

☐Ache, pain in lower abdomen

☐Recent change in sex drive

☐Have had many sexual partners

☐High-impact/ very frequent exercise

☐Crave/ often eat salty foods

☐Hair loss

☐Early graying of hair

☐Significant vaginal discharge

☐Enlarged prostate/ abnormal BPH

☐Impotence/ ED

☐Premature ejaculation

☐Cold body temperature

☐Swelling/ edema in lower body

WOOD/ LIVER/ SPRING

☐Liver disease (cirrhosis, Hepatitis)

☐Frequent alcohol use

☐Gallbladder disease/ stones

☐Eye disorder

☐Dry skin and/or hair

☐Dizziness/ Vertigo

☐Fibromyalgia

☐Headache/ Migraine

☐Frequent sighing or burping

☐Tightness or pain in ribs and/or chest

☐Very tight tendons and ligaments

☐Alternating constipation and diarrhea

☐Spider veins/ varicose veins

☐Tremor disorder/ Parkinson's

☐Muscle spasms

☐Abnormal fingernails (dry, ridged, dark)

☐Seizure disorder/ epilepsy

☐Use of prescription drugs

☐Use of recreational drugs

☐Hormonal birth control (The Pill, IUD)

☐Often irritable, angry or short-tempered

☐Difficulty making decisions

☐Experience long-term, chronic stress

☐Menstrual Cramping

☐Uterine Fibroids or Ovarian Cysts

☐Premenstrual syndrome (PMS)

☐Prior surgery/ operation

☐Bitter taste in mouth

☐Jaundice

☐Swelling or pain of genitals

☐Any of the above "Wood" symptoms are aggravated by stress

About the author

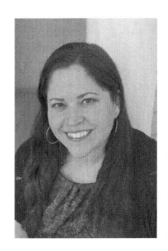

Christine Grisham, Dipl. OM., L.Ac., CMT, MA is the owner of Community Garden Acupuncture in San Diego, California (www.cgacu.com). Her specialties are Japanese style meridian acupuncture, endocrine disorders, chronic diseases, pain management, and end-of-life care. She is a graduate of the Masters of Science in Traditional Oriental Medicine program at Pacific College of Oriental Medicine (PCOM) in San Diego. Christine also holds a Masters of Arts in Public Policy from the Humphrey Institute at the University of Minnesota, and a Bachelors of Arts in Sociology from DePaul University.

Made in the USA
San Bernardino, CA
18 November 2015